Kathryn Quina, PhD
Laura S. Brown, PhD
Editors

Trauma and Dissociation in Convicted Offenders: Gender, Science, and Treatment Issues

Trauma and Dissociation in Convicted Offenders: Gender, Science, and Treatment Issues has been co-published simultaneously as *Journal of Trauma & Dissociation*, Volume 8, Number 2 2007.

*Pre-publication
REVIEWS,
COMMENTARIES,
EVALUATIONS . . .*

"REPRESENTS A MAJOR AD-VANCE for alerting professionals in corrections, mental health and the law about the extensive impact of trauma and dissociation on the lives of offenders. Leading experts provide theoretical, empirical and clinical perspectives for understanding how childhood trauma and dissociative patterns of responding are related to a wide range of problems often encountered in this population, such as substance abuse, HIV risk behaviors, domestic violence perpetration and sex offending. . . . This COMPREHENSIVE volume leaves the reader with a markedly deepened capacity for understanding and more effectively working with convicted offenders. . . . AN INVALUABLE RESOURCE FOR BOTH NOVICE AND VETERAN PROFESSIONALS."

Steven N. Gold, PhD
*Professor
Center for Psychological Studies
Director
Trauma Resolution & Integration
Program (TRIP)
Nova Southeastern University
Fort Lauderdale*

More pre-publication
REVIEWS, COMMENTARIES, EVALUATIONS . . .

"IMPORTANT. . . . In chapters ranging from dissociation and memory in convicted sex offenders to conducting research in prison settings, the editors present useful chapters for all those interested in the effects of trauma on the human psyche and our society. . . . A BRAVE AND PATH BLAZING BOOK, and I hope there are many more to follow."

Pamela Birrell, PhD
Senior Instructor
Psychology Department
University of Oregon, Eugene

"ADDS an important voice to the chorus calling for a change in the way we understand and respond. . . . A NEW VISION OF THE INCARCERATED AS TRAUMA SURVIVORS, women and men coping in similar and different ways, often through dissociation, with the untreated sequela of childhood abuse. . . . MAKES IMPORTANT CONTRIBUTIONS. . . . Provides important focus on the status variables, particularly gender."

Nancy L. Baker, PhD, ABPP
Diplomate in Forensic Psychology
School of Psychology
Fielding Graduate University

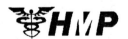

The Haworth Medical Press®
The Haworth Maltreatment & Trauma Press®
Imprints of The Haworth Press, Inc.

Trauma and Dissociation in Convicted Offenders: Gender, Science, and Treatment Issues

Trauma and Dissociation in Convicted Offenders: Gender, Science, and Treatment Issues has been co-published simultaneously as *Journal of Trauma & Dissociation*, Volume 8, Number 2 2007.

Monographic Separates from the *Journal of Trauma & Dissociation*

For additional information on these and other Haworth Press titles, including descriptions, tables of contents, reviews, and prices, use the QuickSearch catalog at http://www.HaworthPress.com.

Trauma and Dissociation in Convicted Offenders: Gender, Science, and Treatment Issues, edited by Kathryn Quina, PhD, and Laura S. Brown, PhD (Vol. 8, No. 2, 2007). *A multifaceted examination at the connection between trauma and the likelihood of being a convicted offender.*

Exploring Dissociation: Definitions, Development and Cognitive Correlates, edited by Anne P. DePrince, PhD, and Lisa DeMarni Cromer, PhD (Vol. 7, No. 4, 2006). *A comprehensive overview of the development and conceptualization of dissociation using classic psychological theories of attachment, learning and memory, attention, and intergenerational transmission of trauma, including innovative models and directions for assessment, treatment, and research.*

Acute Reactions to Trauma and Psychotherapy: A Multidisciplinary and International Perspective, edited by Etzel Cardeña, PhD, and Kristin Croyle, PhD (Vol. 6, No. 2, 2005). *"COMPREHENSIVE. INFORMATIVE. . . . CONCISE AND WELL WRITTEN. . . . A wonderful introduction to a summary of current knowledge about acute stress reactions. . . . A USEFUL RESOURCE FOR GRADUATE STUDENTS as well as for trauma and other mental health researchers and practitioners. . . . Covers a wide range of relevant issues, including vulnerabilities and risk factors, diagnosis, effects of acute stress reactions on the brain, treatment, the role of coping, and peritraumatic dissociation. The research reported here crosses a range of potentially traumatic events and experiences such as house fires, terrorist attacks, and burns." (Laurie Anne Pearlman, PhD, Co-Director, Traumatic Stress Institute/Center for Adult & Adolescent Psychotherapy LLC)*

Trauma and Sexuality: The Effects of Childhood Sexual, Physical, and Emotional Abuse on Sexual Identity and Behavior, edited by James A. Chu, MD, and Elizabeth S. Bowman, MD (Vol. 3, No. 4, 2002). *Examines the effects of childhood trauma on sexual orientation and behavior.*

Trauma and Dissociation in Convicted Offenders: Gender, Science, and Treatment Issues

Kathryn Quina, PhD
Laura S. Brown, PhD
Editors

Trauma and Dissociation in Convicted Offenders: Gender, Science, and Treatment Issues has been co-published simultaneously as *Journal of Trauma & Dissociation*, Volume 8, Number 2 2007.

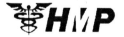

The Haworth Medical Press®
The Haworth Maltreatment & Trauma Press®
Imprints of The Haworth Press, Inc.

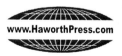

www.HaworthPress.com

Published by

The Haworth Medical Press®, 10 Alice Street, Binghamton, NY 13904-1580 USA

The Haworth Medical Press® is an imprint of The Haworth Press, Inc., 10 Alice Street, Binghamton, NY 13904-1580 USA.

Trauma and Dissociation in Convicted Offenders: Gender, Science, and Treatment Issues has been co-published simultaneously as *Journal of Trauma & Dissociation*, Volume 8, Number 2 2007.

The development, preparation, and publication of this work has been undertaken with great care. However, the publisher, employees, editors, and agents of The Haworth Press and all imprints of The Haworth Press, Inc., including The Haworth Medical Press® and Pharmaceutical Products Press®, are not responsible for any errors contained herein or for consequences that may ensue from use of materials or information contained in this work. With regard to case studies, identities and circumstances of individuals discussed herein have been changed to protect confidentiality. Any resemblance to actual persons, living or dead, is entirely coincidental.

The Haworth Press is committed to the dissemination of ideas and information according to the highest standards of intellectual freedom and the free exchange of ideas. Statements made and opinions expressed in this publication do not necessarily reflect the views of the Publisher, Directors, management, or staff of The Haworth Press, Inc., or an endorsement by them.

Library of Congress Cataloging-in-Publication Data

Trauma and dissociation in convicted offenders : gender, science, and treatment issues / Kathryn Quina, Laura S. Brown, editors.
    p. ; cm.
    "Co-published simultaneously as Journal of Trauma & Dissociation, Volume 8, Number 2 2007".
    Includes bibliographical references and index.
    ISBN 978-0-7890-3328-4 (hard cover : alk. paper)
    1. Prisoners–Mental health. 2. Women prisoners–Mental health. 3. Female offenders–Mental health. 4. Post-traumatic stress disorder. 5. Dissociative disorders. 6. Dual diagnosis. 7. Prison psychology. I. Quina, Kathryn. II. Brown, Laura S. III. Journal of trauma & dissociation.
    [DNLM: 1. Stress Disorders, Post-Traumatic. 2. Dissociative Disorders. 3. Prisoners–psychology. 4. Women–psychology. W1 JO966PK v.8 no.2 2007 / WM 170 T7767 2007]
    RC451.4.P68T67 2007
    616.890086′927–dc22
                                                                                    2007025271

The HAWORTH PRESS, Inc.
Abstracting, Indexing & Outward Linking
PRINT and ELECTRONIC BOOKS & JOURNALS

This section provides you with a list of major indexing & abstracting services and other tools for bibliographic access. That is to say, each service began covering this periodical during the the year noted in the right column. Most Websites which are listed below have indicated that they will either post, disseminate, compile, archive, cite or alert their own Website users with research-based content from this work. (This list is as current as the copyright date of this publication.)

Abstracting, Website/Indexing Coverage . . . . Year When Coverage Began

- *(IBR) International Bibliography of Book Reviews on the Humanities and Social Sciences (Thomson)* <http://www.saur.de> **2006**

- *(IBZ) International Bibliography of Periodical Literature on the Humanitities and Social Sciences (Thomson)* <http://www.saur.de> **2001**

- ***Academic Search Premier (EBSCO)*** <http://search.ebscohost.com> **2006**

- ***EMBASE Excerpta Medica (Elsevier)*** <http://www.elsevier.nl> **2000**

- ***EMBASE.com (The Power of EMBASE + MEDLINE Combined) (Elsevier)*** <http://www.embase.com> **2000**

- ***MEDLINE (National Library of Medicine)*** <http://www.nlm.nih.gov> **2005**

- ***Psychological Abstracts (PsycINFO)*** <http://www.apa.org> . . . **2001**

- ***PubMed*** <http://www.ncbi.nlm.nih.gov/pubmed/> **2005**

- *Academic Source Premier (EBSCO)* <http://search.ebscohost.com> **2007**

- *Biology Digest (in print & online)* <http://www.infotoday.com> . . **2000**

(continued)

(continued)

(continued)

Bibliographic Access

- ***Cabell's Directory of Publishing Opportunities in Psychology*** *<http://www.cabells.com>*

- ***MediaFinder*** *<http://www.mediafinder.com/>*

- ***Ulrich's Periodicals Directory: The Global Source for Periodicals Information Since 1932*** *<http://www.bowkerlink.com>*

Special Bibliographic Notes related to special journal issues (separates) and indexing/abstracting:

- indexing/abstracting services in this list will also cover material in any "separate" that is co-published simultaneously with Haworth's special thematic journal issue or DocuSerial. Indexing/abstracting usually covers material at the article/chapter level.
- monographic co-editions are intended for either non-subscribers or libraries which intend to purchase a second copy for their circulating collections.
- monographic co-editions are reported to all jobbers/wholesalers/approval plans. The source journal is listed as the "series" to assist the prevention of duplicate purchasing in the same manner utilized for books-in-series.
- to facilitate user/access services all indexing/abstracting services are encouraged to utilize the co-indexing entry note indicated at the bottom of the first page of each article/chapter/contribution.
- this is intended to assist a library user of any reference tool (whether print, electronic, online, or CD-ROM) to locate the monographic version if the library has purchased this version but not a subscription to the source journal.
- individual articles/chapters in any Haworth publication are also available through the Haworth Document Delivery Service (HDDS).

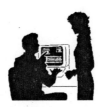

As part of Haworth's continuing commitment to better serve our library patrons, we are proud to be working with the following electronic services:

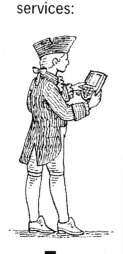

AGGREGATOR SERVICES

EBSCOhost

Ingenta

J-Gate

Minerva

OCLC FirstSearch FirstSearch .

Oxmill

SwetsWise SwetsWise

LINK RESOLVER SERVICES

1Cate (Openly Informatics)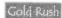

ChemPort
(American Chemical Society) ChemPort®

CrossRef

Gold Rush (Coalliance) Gold Rush

LinkOut (PubMed) LinkOut.

LINKplus (Atypon)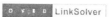

LinkSolver (Ovid)

LinkSource with A-to-Z (EBSCO)

Resource Linker (Ulrich)

SerialsSolutions (ProQuest) SerialsSolutions

SFX (Ex Libris) S·F·X

Sirsi Resolver (SirsiDynix) SirsiDynix

Tour (TDnet) TOUR

Vlink (Extensity, formerly Geac) extensity

WebBridge (Innovative Interfaces) WebBridge

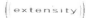

Trauma and Dissociation in Convicted Offenders: Gender, Science, and Treatment Issues

CONTENTS

ABOUT THE EDITORS

Kathryn Quina, PhD, earned her doctorate in 1973 at the University of Georgia, and is Professor of Psychology and Women's Studies at the University of Rhode Island, where she has won several teaching and service awards. For over 30 years, her research has examined the sequelae of childhood trauma in its various forms. She coauthored *Childhood Trauma and HIV: Women at Risk* and *Sexual Assault and Harassment: A Guide to Helping Survivors*. Her current research examines the role of childhood trauma in the life paths of incarcerated women. Her other interests include pedagogy and academic equity; she co-edited *Teaching Gender and Multicultural Awareness: Resources for the Psychology Classroom* and *Career Strategies for Women in Academe: Arming Athena*. Dr. Quina received the Distinguished Publication Award, the Christine Ladd Franklin Award for professional service, and the Florence Denmark Mentoring Award from the Association for Women in Psychology, and is a Fellow of the American Psychological Association (Divisions 2, 9, and 35).

Laura S. Brown, PhD, earned her doctorate in clinical psychology in 1977 from Southern Illinois University, and since 1979 has been in the independent practice of feminist therapy and forensic psychology in Seattle. She has published extensively on topics of feminist therapy theory, ethics, and practice, on forensic assessment of trauma, trauma and cultural competence, and trauma and memory. Her awards include two Distinguished Publications Awards from the Association for Women in Psychology, the Sarah Haley Award from the International Society for Traumatic Stress Studies, the Carolyn Wood Sherif Memorial Award from the Society for the Psychology of Women, and the Award for Distinguished Professional Contributions to Public Service from the American Psychological Association. Her two videos on trauma treatment are produced and published by APA's video series. A Fellow of the American Psychological Association and the Association for Psychological Science, she is past-president of APA's Division 35 and 44, and of the Washington State Psychological Association. In 2006 she founded the Fremont Community Therapy Project, a low-fee clinic offering psychotherapy and psychological assessment to the greater Seattle area and training opportunities for doctoral students in psychology. Currently she is the Director of the Fremont Community Therapy Project, Seattle, Washington. Dr. Brown presently serves on the editorial boards of six journals, and is the web editor for APA Division 56 (Trauma Psychology). In 1989 she was the expert witness for women prisoners in Washington State in the landmark prisoner's rights case Jordan v. Gardner, which protects women prisoners in Washington from intimate pat-searches by male corrections staff. She is a Diplomate in Clinical Psychology of the American Board of Professionial Psychology, a Fellow of the Association for Psychologicail Science, and a Fellow of APA in Divisions 9, 12, 29, 35, 42, 43, 44, 45, 46, and 56.

Introduction

According to the most recent statistics, over two million men and women were incarcerated in prisons or jails in the United States, a number that has increased steadily since 1986 (Bureau of Justice Statistics (BJS), 2005). One in 10 is female, and rates of incarceration for women have consistently risen faster than those for men. Black and Hispanic men and women are disproportionately overrepresented among inmates; Blacks and Hispanic men are 7 and 2.6 times more likely to be incarcerated than Euro-Americans relative to their representation in the non-prison populations. In 1997, the latest year for which estimates are provided by BJS, approximately 9% of the Black population and 2% of the white population were under some form of correctional supervision; across race, this included 5% of men and 1% of women.

Within the incarcerated population there are high rates of substance abuse and mental illness, and these problems tend to co-occur. According to BJS, between 42 and 49% of prisoners meet DSM-IV criteria for both mental health problems and substance dependence or abuse; in addition, more than 20% meet criteria for drug problems and 15% for mental health problems alone (James & Glaze, 2006). Over a quarter of prisoners nationally report that they were using drugs at the time they committed their offense (Mumola & Karberg, 2006). National surveys also reveal that 45-63% of male and 60-75% of female inmates had met DSM-IV criteria for mental health problems in the previous year. About 20% of men, and 40% of women, had seen a mental health professional or been diagnosed by one during the previous year, and over 20% of all inmates had been prescribed psychotropic medications (James & Glaze, 2006).

[Haworth co-indexing entry note]: "Introduction." Quina, Kathryn, and Laura S. Brown. Co-published simultaneously in *Journal of Trauma & Dissociation* (The Haworth Medical Press, an imprint of The Haworth Press, Inc.) Vol. 8, No. 2, 2007, pp. 1-7; and: *Trauma and Dissociation in Convicted Offenders: Gender, Science, and Treatment Issues* (ed: Kathryn Quina, and Laura S. Brown) The Haworth Medical Press, an imprint of The Haworth Press, Inc., 2007, pp. 1-7. Single or multiple copies of this article are available for a fee from The Haworth Document Delivery Service [1-800-HAWORTH, 9:00 a.m. - 5:00 p.m. (EST). E-mail address: docdelivery@haworthpress.com].

Available online at http://jtd.haworthpress.com
doi:10.1300/J229v08n02_01

Trauma consistently appears in conjunction with these mental health and drug abuse statistics. The only national study of inmates (Harlow, 1999) found that nearly 50% of the women and 10% of the men had experienced some form of abuse prior to being incarcerated. Of these, 23-37% of women and 6-14% of men reported sexual abuse prior to the age of 18. Other studies, however, find rates as high as 73% among females (Chesney-Lind & Shelden, 1992), and 59% among males (Johnson, et al., 2005), involved in the criminal justice system. Furthermore, women who were abused as children are much more likely to be abused after they turn 18, mostly by intimate partners or family members (e.g., Whitmire, Harlow, Quina, & Morokoff, 1999).

These are individuals who are most likely to be described as experiencing what Herman first described as "Complex Trauma" (Herman, 1992), a combination of post-traumatic factors in which damage to attachment and self-systems, in addition to more usual post-traumatic changes to biological and psychological functioning, are likely to be present. Persons with complex trauma are likely to have serious challenges with affect regulation and self-soothing, are more likely to utilize dissociation of some form as a survival strategy, and in general experience difficulties across all aspects of functioning. Harlow's (1999) analyses and research with male (Johnson et al., 2005) and female offenders (e.g., Pimlott-Kubiak, 2003) also revealed that both men and women reporting prior abuse were more likely to use illegal drugs and alcohol regularly, similar to other survivors of complex trauma (Briere & Scott, 2006), among whom substance abuse is a condition commonly co-morbid with PTSD and complex trauma. Violent crimes, including homicide, sexual assault and robbery, were more prevalent among men and women reporting prior abuse (although these crimes were far more likely to have been committed by men than by women).

This volume presents a multifaceted look at the individuals behind statistics such as these, with literature reviews, case studies, results of empirical studies, models for intervention, and issues for researchers and clinicians working within a correctional system with survivors of complex trauma who manifest with a myriad of post-traumatic and dissociative symptom pictures. Our primary goal is to inform and educate readers engaged in research, therapy, education, and public policy about the "pathways to prison." However, we entered this with another, more personal hope: that in reading these articles, each of us gains a greater understanding of the men and women who are arguably the individuals most affected by trauma in our society, and perhaps makes a personal commitment to changing the ways in which we treat them for the better.

The articles have been framed around issues of trauma and dissociation, in line with the research data and clinical experiences of experts working with inmates. The authors have tended to focus on the trauma of childhood sexual abuse (CSA), perhaps because its effects are so strongly implicated in risk for involvement with the criminal justice system (Adams, 2002; Browne, Miller, & Maguin, 1999), difficulties during incarceration (Neller, Denney, Pietz, & Thomlinson, 2006), and recidivism (Hochstetler, Murphy, & Simons, 2004). Particularly when the abuse is severe and perpetrated by multiple or familial repeat abusers, CSA has been linked to a wide range of negative outcomes, including poor health and mental health, disrupted relationships, and self-destructive behaviors. Although the minority of persons with complex trauma enter a trajectory into the criminal justice system, being multiply and repeatedly subjected to maltreatment and neglect early in development is one certain way to increase an individual's risk for residing in a prison at some point in their life (Boney-McCoy & Finkelhor, 1995; Gilligan, 1996).

Among the strategies for coping with severe, unavoidable abuse is dissociation in its many forms. Dissociative coping strategies are means of not knowing, not feeling, and not being present with intolerable physical and emotional pain. Dissociation is a common component of the complex trauma response (van der Kolk et al., 1996), and has been identified as an issue for inmates with CSA histories (Dietrich, 2003). Complex trauma response is not limited to the DSM-IV-TR category of dissociative disorders, but rather inhabits a broader spectrum of coping strategies. Furthermore, it is our belief that one behavior serving as a dissociative coping strategy is substance use. As noted in the national BJS analyses (James & Glaze, 2006), higher rates of alcohol and drug use have been observed in survivors of CSA as well as child physical abuse and other traumatic experiences, and Post Traumatic Stress Disorder and Substance Use Disorder are known to co-occur (e.g., Battle, Zlotnick, Najavits, Gutierrez, & Winsor, 2003). This is true for people both in and out of the prison system; what we know is that substance abuse is becoming increasingly the most direct path to prison, with the majority of new women inmates in the state of Washington, for example, coming into the system in the wake of drug-related offenses (John Haroian, personal communication, July, 2006).

CSA in both women and men is also a risk factor for entering prostitution, an activity which is criminalized in this country and thus an entry-level crime for a number of survivors. Prostitution concatenates with substance abuse, with many street prostitutes working to obtain money for drugs, and many put at risk of more serious criminal offenses due to their associations with their suppliers and their procurers (e.g., Graham & Wish, 1994).

CSA and other traumas occur within a system of advantages or disadvantages which can reduce or enhance their deleterious effects. Among these are status variables–primarily income, race, and gender (Figueira-McDonough & Sarri, 2002)–and individual challenges such as disability, education, job training, and family environment. Neurological problems, including those caused by traumatic experiences, may also be a factor (Brewer-Smyth, 2004). There is no universal victim, nor a universal criminal; to intervene appropriately we need to appreciate the diversity of individual inmates and their experiences.

Each of the articles in this volume builds a strong case for the connections among early traumas and other problematic sequelae. The conclusion one is compelled to draw, from the literatures reviewed and the new information presented in the articles in this volume, is that we can, and should stop the cycles of violence, criminal activities, substance abuse, and recidivism which create of our prisons one of the largest institutions housing trauma survivors. However, such trauma-focused and CSA-aware interventions are rare in the corrections system. After incarceration, only 11% of inmates report receiving mental health services and only 15% participated in drug treatment, while another 35-40% participated in other drug use-related programs (James & Glaze, 2006). Since juvenile offending is often a precursor of adult incarceration, it is essential to transform both juvenile and adult systems into places of safety, with opportunities to address and move beyond the devastating effects of trauma.

It is interesting that most of the authors who responded to our call for papers for this volume were working with women offenders. Perhaps this is because of the higher rates of CSA and adult victimization experiences generally reported by women inmates, and the stronger subsequent associations with the crimes for which they are frequently incarcerated, drug use and sex work (Farley & Barkan, 1998; Graham & Wish, 1994). Perhaps it is in recognition of the fact that the impact of CSA falls disproportionately on women and their children, and even more disproportionately on mothers who enter the prison system and their children, who are at risk–especially in foster care or in the care of relatives who were the original source of trauma in the mother's life (e.g., Enos, 2001). Perhaps this is because we tend to fear women offenders less, presuming them less violent, and thus are more likely to study them (a statistically accurate assumption, but in practical terms few who conduct research or therapy in prisons are placed in potentially harmful circumstances). Perhaps it is because women's facilities, which often feature smaller numbers of inmates and less overcrowding, have been more open to the additional disruptions caused by research and programming.

Whatever the reasons, it is important to consider how the information presented here might relate on a larger scale to incarcerated men, and hopefully some of our readers will be inspired to continue expanding our knowledge and understanding with other populations. Trauma, particularly sexual trauma, is a gendered phenomenon; the traumatized man sees himself as weak, and may act out criminally as a defense against being seen as vulnerable. It is possible that there are higher rates of trauma in the lives of male inmates than known, given the manner in which being a trauma survivor is gendered, and the impact of that phenomenon on self-report.

Our professional careers in academia/research (KQ) and academia/ therapy (LSB) have been infused with and informed by feminist approaches (Brown, 1994; Freyd & Quina, 2000). It can be no different in our work related to corrections. As such, we encourage our readers to consider how gender, social class, and cultural histories of trauma have intersected in the lives of many incarcerated people, rendering them a group of people whose trauma response is particularly complex and problematic. In assembling this volume, we pay tribute to the experts "in the trenches" who have brilliantly laid out the case for understanding prisoners, in particular women prisoners, as an underserved and marginalized group of individuals (e.g., Chesney-Lind, 1998; Fine & Carney, 2001; Harden & Hill, 1998). Women and men in prison have broken the law. They are also survivors of trauma whose distress and behavioral dysfunctions should be of interest to all professionals concerned with the topics of trauma and dissociation.

Kathryn Quina, PhD
Department of Psychology
University of Rhode Island
Kingston, RI 02881

Laura S. Brown, PhD
Director, Fremont Community Therapy Project
Seattle, WA 98103

REFERENCES

Adams, J. (2002). Child abuse: The fundamental issue in forensic clinical practice. *International Journal of Offender Therapy and Comparative Criminology, 46*(6), 729-733.

Battle, C. L., Zlotnick, C., Najavits, L. M., Gutierrez, M., & Winsor, C. (2003). Post traumatic stress disorder and substance use disorder among incarcerated women. In P. Ouimette & P. J. Brown (Eds.), *Trauma and substance abuse: Causes, consequences, and treatment of comorbid disorders* (pp. 209-225). Washington, DC: American Psychological Association.

Boney-McCoy, S., & Finkelhor, D. (1995). Psycho-social sequelae of violent victimization in a national youth sample. *Journal of Consulting and Clinical Psychology, 63*, 726-736.

Brewer-Smyth, K. (2004). Women behind bars: Could neurobiological correlates of past physical and sexual abuse contribute to criminal behavior? *Health Care for Women International, 25*, 835-852.

Briere, J. & Scott, C. (2006) *Principles of trauma therapy: A guide to symptoms, evaluation, and treatment.* Thousand Oaks, CA: Sage Publications.

Brown, A., Miller, B., & Maguin, E. (1999). Prevalence and severity of lifetime physical and sexual victimization among incarcerated women. *International Journal of Law & Psychiatry, 22*, 301-322.

Brown, L. S. (1994). *Subversive dialogues: Theory in feminist therapy.* New York: Basic Books.

Bureau of Justice Statistics (2005). *Prison statistics.* Retrieved 10/1/06 from http://www.ojp.usdoj.gov/bjs/prisons.htm.

Chesney-Lind, M. (1997). *The female offender: Girls, women, and crime.* Thousand Oaks, CA: Sage Publications.

Chesney, Lind, M., & Shelden, R. G. (1992). *Girls, delinquency and juvenile justice.* Pacific Grove, CA: Brooks/Cole.

Enos, S. (2001). *Mothering from the inside: Parenting in a women's prison.* Albany, NY: State University of New York Press.

Farley, M., & Barkan, H. (1998). Prostitution, violence, and Posttraumatic Stress Disorder. *Women's Health, 27*, 37-49.

Figueira-McDonough, J., & Sarri, R. C. (Eds.). (2002). *Women at the margins: Neglect, punishment, and resistance.* Binghamton, NY: The Haworth Press.

Fine, M., & Carney, S. (2001). Women, gender, and the law: Toward a feminist rethinking of responsibility. In R. Unger (Ed.), *Handbook of psychology and gender.* New York: McMillan Publishers, 388-409.

Freyd, J. J., & Quina, K. (2000). Feminist ethics in the practice of science: The contested memory controversy as example. In M. Brabeck (Ed.), *Practicing ethics in feminist psychology* (pp. 101-124). Washington, DC: American Psychological Association.

Gilligan, J. (1996). *Violence: Reflections on a national epidemic.* New York: Random House.

Graham, N., & Wish, E. D. (1994). Drug use among female arrestees: Onset, patterns, and relationships to prostitution. *Journal of Drug Issues, 24*, 315-329.

Harden, J., & Hill, M. (Eds.). (1998). *Breaking the rules: Women in prison and feminist therapy.* New York: The Haworth Press.

Harlow, C. W. (1999). *Prior abuse reported by inmates and probationers.* Retrieved 10/1/06 from http://www.ojp.usdoj.gov/bjs/pub/pdf/parip.pdf.

Herman, J. (1997). *Trauma and Recovery: The Aftermath of Violence–from Domestic Abuse to Political Terror.* New York: Basic Books.

Hochstetler, A., Murphy, D. S., & Simons, R. L. (2004). Damaged goods: Exploring predictors of distress in prison inmates. *Crime & Delinquency, 50*(3), 436-457.

James, D. J., & Glaze, L. E. (2006). Mental health problems of prison and jail inmates. Retrieved 10/1/06 from http://www.ojp.usdoj.gov/bjs/pub/pdf/mhppji.pdf.

Johnson, R. J., Ross, M. W., Taylor, W. C., Williams, M. L., Carvajal, R. I., & Peters, R. J. (2005). A history of drug use and child sexual abuse among incarcerated males in a county jail. *Substance Use and Misuse, 40,* 211-229.

Mumola, C. J., & Karberg, J. C. (2006). Drug dependence, state and federal prisoners, 2004. Retrieved 10/1/06 from http://www.ojp.usdoj.gov/bjs/pub/pdf/dudsfp04.pdf.

Neller, D. J., Denney, R. L., Pietz, C. A., & Thomlinson, R. P. (2006). The relationship between trauma and violence in a jail inmate sample. *Journal of Interpersonal Violence, 21*(9), 1234-1241.

Pimlott-Kubiak, S. M. (2003). Social location and cumulative adversity in multiply traumatized women. *Dissertation Abstracts International: Section B: The Sciences and Engineering, 63*(10-B), 4818.

van der Kolk, B. A., Pelcovitz, D., Roth, S., Mandel, F. S., McFarlane, A., & Herman, J. L. (1996). Dissociation, somatization, and affect dysregulation: The complexity of adaptation to trauma. *American Journal of Psychiatry, 153,* 83-93.

Whitmire, L., Harlow, L. L., Quina, K., & Morokoff, P. J. (1999). *Childhood trauma and HIV: Women at risk.* New York: Taylor & Francis.

doi:10.1300/J229v08n02_01

The Relationship
of Lifetime Polysubstance Dependence
to Trauma Exposure, Symptomatology,
and Psychosocial Functioning
in Incarcerated Women
with Comorbid PTSD
and Substance Use Disorder

Dawn M. Salgado, PhD
Kristen J. Quinlan, PhD
Caron Zlotnick, PhD

Dawn M. Salgado is affiliated with the Department of Psychology, University of Rhode Island, Kingston, Rhode Island.

Kristen J. Quinlan is affiliated with Rhode Island Department of Mental Health, Retardation and Hospitals, and Department of Psychology, University of Rhode Island, Kingston, Rhode Island.

Caron Zlotnick is Director of Behavioral Medicine Research at Women and Infants Hospital, and Associate Professor, Department of Psychiatry and Human Behavior, Brown Medical School, Butler Hospital, Providence, Rhode Island.

Address correspondence to: Caron Zlotnick, Brown Medical School/Butler Hospital, 345 Blackstone Boulevard, Providence, RI 02906 (E-mail: CZlotnick@butler.org).

This work was supported by National Institute of Drug Abuse (DA139359) and the National Institute of Justice (#95166).

[Haworth co-indexing entry note]: "The Relationship of Lifetime Polysubstance Dependence to Trauma Exposure, Symptomatology, and Psychosocial Functioning in Incarcerated Women with Comorbid PTSD and Substance Use Disorder." Salgado, Dawn M., Kristen J. Quinlan, and Caron Zlotnick. Co-published simultaneously in *Journal of Trauma & Dissociation* (The Haworth Medical Press, an imprint of The Haworth Press, Inc.) Vol. 8, No. 2, 2007, pp. 9-26; and: *Trauma and Dissociation in Convicted Offenders: Gender, Science, and Treatment Issues* (ed: Kathryn Quina, and Laura S. Brown) The Haworth Medical Press, an imprint of The Haworth Press, Inc., 2007, pp. 9-26. Single or multiple copies of this article are available for a fee from The Haworth Document Delivery Service [1-800-HAWORTH, 9:00 a.m. - 5:00 p.m. (EST). E-mail address: docdelivery@haworthpress.com].

Available online at http://jtd.haworthpress.com
doi:10.1300/J229v08n02_02

SUMMARY. There is a dearth of literature examining the relationship between trauma-related experiences, PTSD, and lifetime polysubstance dependence among incarcerated women. A sample of 69 treatment-seeking incarcerated women with current PTSD and comorbid substance use disorder (PTSD-SUD) were recruited from a northeastern state medium-security prison. Women with lifetime polysubstance dependence (PTSD-SUD/LPD; *n* = 33) were compared to women with no lifetime polysubstance dependence (PTSD-SUD only; *n* = 36) across a range of features: trauma characteristics (e.g., number of traumas, type of trauma), associated symptoms (e.g., dissociation, anxiety), severity of substance use and psychosocial functioning. Women with PTSD and lifetime polysubstance dependence reported greater severity of drug and alcohol use, increased exposure to traumatic events (i.e., general disasters, crime-related events), and increased prevalence of PTSD-related symptoms (i.e., derealization, survivor guilt). Trends also suggest that PTSD-SUD/LPD women are more likely to experience dissociation, anxiety, and sexual problems than PTSD-SUD respondents. Treatment-related implications are discussed. doi:10.1300/J229v08n02_02 *[Article copies available for a fee from The Haworth Document Delivery Service: 1-800- HAWORTH. E-mail address: <docdelivery@haworthpress.com> Website: <http://www. HaworthPress.com>* © 2007 by The Haworth Press, Inc. All rights reserved.]

KEYWORDS. Polysubstance dependence, PTSD-SUD, incarcerated women

DISORDER

Previous research with community samples suggests that women with current Posttraumatic Stress Disorder (PTSD) are at greater risk for comorbid Substance Use Disorders (SUD) compared to women without PTSD (Helzer, Robins, & McEvoy, 1987; Kilpatrick Resnick, Saunders, & Best, 1996; Kulka et al., 1990; Ouimette, Wolfe, & Chrestman, 1996; Najavits, Weiss, & Shaw, 1997; Zlotnick, Bruce, Weisberg, Shea et al., 2003). Additionally, women with comorbid PTSD and SUD experience a greater number of traumatic events in childhood, are more likely to have experienced childhood sexual and physical abuse, and are more likely to have experienced adult sexual assault than women with a primary diagnosis of substance abuse alone (Brady, Killeen, Saladin, Dansky, & Becker, 1994; Ouimette et al., 1996). In one sample of female primary care patients with PTSD, Zlotnick et al. (2003) found that those with comorbid SUD experienced prolonged episodes of PTSD when compared to those without SUD. Similarly, others (Brady et al., 1994; Brown & Wolfe, 1994; Cottler, Compton, Mager, Spitznagel, & Janker, 1992; Dansky, Roitzsch, Brady, & Saladin, 1995; Druley & Pashko, 1988; Goldenberg et al., 1995; Ouimette, Ahrens, Moos, & Finney, 1997) have noted that individuals with comorbid PTSD and substance dependence are generally found to have a poorer prognosis, related to more severe drug use, increased health-related problems, and more illegal activity, when compared to those individuals with PTSD or substance dependence exclusively.

Although studies have documented that comorbid PTSD and SUD is related to psychiatric, medical and social morbidity, few studies have examined comorbid PTSD-SUD among female incarcerated populations, a population of women who report high rates of trauma exposure, PTSD, and substance abuse and dependence (Teplin, Abram, & McClelland, 1996). Between 78 to 99% of incarcerated women have experienced at least one traumatic event (Cook, Smith, Tusher, & Raiford, 2005; Jordan Schlenger, Fairbank, & Caddell, 1996; Lake, 1993; Resnick, Kilpatrick, Dansky, Saunders, & Best, 1993; Singer, Bussey, Song, & Lunghofer, 1995), with other research (Cook et al., 2005) suggesting that up to 81% of incarcerated women have been exposed to five or more traumatic events in their lifetime. Specifically, high rates of childhood and adult victimization are common among incarcerated women (American Correctional Association, 1991; Bradley & Davino, 2002; Browne, Miller, & Maguin, 1999; Maeve, 2000; Parsons & Warner-Robbins, 2002; U.S. Department of Justice, 1999), with large-scale studies of this population reporting rates of physical and sexual victimization between 36 and 60% (ACA, 2001; U.S Department of Justice, 1999).

Prevalence rates of PTSD in the female prison population have been less well studied compared to those of SUD. Researchers who have examined prevalence rates have found that rates of PTSD among women prisoners are more than twice the rates of PTSD reported in a community sample of women (Kessler et al., 1995). Among those female jail detainees awaiting trial, Teplin et al. (1996) found that PTSD was the most common disorder diagnosed, besides substance dependence, with prevalence rates of 33.5% for lifetime PTSD and 22.3% for current PTSD. Others (Jordan et al., 1996; Lewis, 2005a, b; Teplin et al., 1996) have reported rates of lifetime prevalence of PTSD among incarcerated women from 30 to 42%, with specific subpopulations of incarcerated women (e.g., HIV-positive) with rates as high as 74.1%.

Previous research has also documented high rates of substance use disorders among incarcerated women (Bradley & Davino, 2002; Covington,

1998; Desjardins, Brochu, & Biron, 1992; Jordan et al., 1996; Peters, Greenbaum, Edens, Carter & Ortiz, 1998; Richie, 2001; U.S. Department of Justice, 1999; Teplin et al., 1996). Incarcerated women are more likely to be involved in crimes related to alcohol or drugs than male inmates and are five to eight times more likely to abuse alcohol, ten times more likely to abuse drugs, and 27 times more likely to use cocaine than women in the general population (Covington, 1998; Desjardins et al., 1992; Jordan et al., 1996; Teplin et al., 1996). Given the high rates of trauma exposure and substance use among incarcerated women, co-occurring PTSD and SUD are common (Zlotnick, 1997). Yet, few studies to date (for example, see Zlotnick et al., 2003) have investigated the prevalence and clinical outcomes of incarcerated women with co-occurring PTSD and SUD.

In response to this lack of research on incarcerated women with comorbid PTSD-SUD, the current study examined differences along a range of clinical correlates in a sample of incarcerated women with and without comorbid lifetime polysubstance dependence, all of whom met criteria for comorbid PTSD and substance use disorder. Unlike substance use dependence, which is based on use of a single drug, lifetime polysubstance dependence is defined as substance use "during the same 12 month period in which the person was repeatedly using at least 3 groups of substances, but no single substance predominated" (DSM-IV, 1995). Previous research with other populations suggests that those individuals with lifetime polysubstance dependence experience more psychological and physical health problems and report increased exposure to traumatic events (e.g., violence, child abuse), increased institutionalization, and increased family instability when compared to those who are alcohol or drug-dependent exclusively or those without substance dependence (Agosti & Levin, 2006; Booth, Sullivan, Koegel, & Burnam, 2002; Cottler et al., 2001; Tomasson & Vaglum, 1998; Triffleman, Marmar, Delucchi, & Ronfeldt, 1995).

Using a sample of incarcerated women with comorbid PTSD and SUD, we seek to add to this literature by examining how individuals with and without lifetime polysubstance dependence differ on trauma characteristics (e.g., number of traumas, type of trauma), trauma-related symptoms (e.g., dissociation, anxiety), severity of alcohol and drug use, and psychosocial functioning (e.g., legal problems, psychiatric difficulties, employment status). By examining these clinical correlates in a sample of incarcerated women, the current study aims to contribute to empirical research concerning polysubstance dependence in a population of women with high levels of psychosocial dysfunction and treatment needs.

METHODS

Participants

Women in a medium security New England prison were recruited to participate in a study examining the efficacy of *Seeking Safety*, a cognitive-behavioral treatment for comorbid PTSD and SUD (Najavits, 2002; Najavits, Weiss, Shaw, & Muenez, 1998; Zlotnick, 2002). To participate in the treatment, women had to meet DSM-IV criteria for PTSD within the last month, meet criteria for substance abuse/dependence disorder one month prior to entering prison, and be primarily English-speaking.

The current study is based on intake data from 77 incarcerated women who were assessed for the treatment study. As shown in Table 1, the majority of the sample identified as White, non-Hispanic (54.5%) followed by African American/Black (19.5%), Hispanic/Latino (13.0%), and Native American (5.2%). Most respondents were over the age of 30 (63.6%) and had graduated from high school (33.8%) or some college level courses (16.9%). In terms of family structure, most women reported either having never married (37.7%) or being separated/divorced (44.2%), and reported having children under the age of 18 (69.4%). Prior to incarceration, most were unemployed (63.6%), although a significant minority was employed on at least a part-time basis (23.4%).

Incarceration information indicated that most of the respondents had a prior conviction (88.3%) and that the average number of previous convictions ranged from a minimum of 1 to a maximum of 50 ($M = 7.03$, $SD = 7.81$). Most respondents had been arrested for misdemeanors (58.4%), and analysis of specific offenses revealed that drug-related offenses were the most common (45.7%), followed by robbery/burglary (17.6%), larceny or theft (14.7%), and fraud (11.8%). Consistent with previous findings (Bradley & Davino, 2002; Richie, 2001; U.S. Department of Justice, 1999), only a minority of women were convicted for violent offenses like assault ($n = 3$, or 8.8%).

Measures

Background information. Respondents were asked to provide general demographic information, including information about ethnicity,

TABLE 1. Demographic Characteristics for Total Sample

	n	%
Race		
White (Non-Hispanic)	42	54.5
Afro-American	15	19.5
Hispanic (Latino)	10	13.0
Native American	4	5.2
Other	6	7.8
Current Age		
Less than 25 years	6	7.8
26-30 years	22	28.6
31-35 years	22	28.6
Greater than 36 years	27	35.1
Educational Attainment		
Less than 8th grade	15	19.5
Some high school	23	29.9
High school graduate or equivalent	26	33.8
Some college/vocational training	13	16.9
Marital Status		
Single, never married	29	37.7
Separated	23	29.9
Divorced	11	14.3
Married	8	10.4
Widowed	5	6.5
Living as married	1	1.3
Children–18 years old or younger[a]		
Yes	34	69.4
No	15	30.6
Pre-Imprisonment Employment		
Full time	13	16.9
Part time	5	6.5
Disability/Retired	8	10.4
Unemployed	49	63.6
Other	2	2.6
First Sentence		
Yes	9	11.7
No	68	88.3
Type of Crime		
Misdemeanor	45	58.4
Felony	32	41.6

	n	%
Nature of Crime Committed[b]		
Drug possession, dealing, other drug-related offense	16	45.7
Robbery/Burglary	6	17.6
Larceny or theft	5	14.7
Fraud	4	11.8
Violent assault	3	8.8
Weapons possession	3	8.8
Stolen property	2	5.9
Negligent manslaughter	1	2.9
Remaining Length of Sentence[a]		
Less than 2 months	3	6.1
3-6 months	33	67.3
6 months to 1 year	10	20.4
Greater than 1 year	3	6.1

Note. [a] Not all respondent data were available; [b]Includes those with specific documented crimes ($n = 34$; categories are not mutually exclusive).

age, religion. Participants were also asked about family structure (e.g., current marital status, the number of children under 18 living in the home), educational level, employment, and income prior to arrest. In addition to general demographics, information was also collected with regard to the type of crime, number of arrests with convictions, and the sentence length.

Clinician-Administered Posttraumatic Stress Disorder Scale (CAPs; Blake et al., 1990; Weathers, Ruscio, & Keane, 1999). Participants were assessed using the Clinician-Administered Posttraumatic Stress Disorder Scale (CAPs), a structured clinical interview that assesses seventeen symptoms of PTSD outlined in DSM-IV (APA, 1994) in adult respondents, including the presence of five associated features related to guilt and dissociation (i.e., guilt, survivor guilt, derealization, depersonalization, and lack of awareness in one's surroundings).

Participants were asked to respond to a series of standardized and follow-up items related to their experience with specific traumatic events and were then asked to rate the intensity of their symptoms (0 = Never to 4 = Daily or almost every day) and the severity of their symptoms (0 = None to 4 = Extreme, incapacitating distress). Total scores, as well as composite scores for each cluster (i.e., re-experiencing, numbing and avoidance, hyperarousal), were calculated for each respondent. The CAPs has demonstrated sound reliability and validity (Blake et al., 1990) and can be used as a screening measure to determine inclusion criteria for interventions or to create a relatively homogenous group in which to compare those who are PTSD positive with those who are PTSD negative (Weathers et al., 1999).

Structured Clinical Interview for Diagnostic and Statistical Manual of Mental Disorders (SCID; 4th ed.; *DSM-IV;* First, Spitzer, Gibbon, & Williams, 1997). The substance use disorder module from the Structured Clinical Interview for the Diagnostic and Statistical Manual of Mental Disorders was administered to determine lifetime and current (i.e., past month prior to incarceration) alcohol or drug use dependence, as well as polysubstance dependence.

Trauma History Questionnaire (THQ; Green, 1996). The Trauma History Questionnaire (THQ) is a 23-item self-report instrument used to assess a participant's history of exposure to traumatic events related to crime (e.g., mugging, robbery), sexual or physical assault (e.g., unwanted sexual contact, attacked with weapon) or general disasters (e.g., accidents, natural disasters, serious injury). Participants were asked to indicate lifetime exposure to a specific event ($0 = $ no, $1 = $ yes), the number of times the event occurred ($0 = $ never, $1 = $ once, $2 = $ 2-10 times, $3 = $ 10-20 times, $4 = $ 20 or more times, $5 = $ too many times to remember, or $6 = $ cannot remember how many times) and the age that the trauma was first experienced.

Trauma Symptom Checklist (TCS; Briere & Runtz, 1989). The Trauma Symptom Checklist (TCS) is a 40-item measure examining the frequency in which specific symptomatology is experienced by the respondent. Items are rated on a 4-point scale ($0 = $ Never to $3 = $ Very Often) to create a total scale score, as well as six subscales: anxiety, depression, dissociation, sexual abuse trauma index, sexual problems, and sleep disturbance. Example symptoms include "feeling tense all the time," "feeling that things are 'unreal'," and experiencing "restless sleep."

Addiction Severity Index (ASI; McLellan, Kushner, Metzger, Peters et al., 1992; McGahan, Griffith, Parente, & McLellan, 1986). The Addiction Severity Index (ASI) is a clinician administered, semi-structured interview used to assess the severity of recent (i.e., 30 days prior to incarceration) problems in seven functional areas: medical, employment, alcohol, drug, legal, family/social, and psychiatric. Participants are asked to indicate the degree to which they have been troubled by problems in each of these functional areas, and the interviewer also assigns a severity rating for each of the functional areas, indicating the interviewer's assessment of the participant's need for treatment. The ASI has been used as a standard assessment and diagnostic tool for determining substance use dependence with composite scores ranging from 0.00 (no problem) to 1.00 (greatest severity).

RESULTS

Sixty-nine respondents of the total 77 (89.6%) with SUD in the month prior to incarceration also met criteria for current PTSD. Of those 69 respondents with current PTSD, 47.8% ($n = 33$) of respondents also reported lifetime polysubstance dependence (PTSD-SUD/LPD) and the other 52.2% ($n = 36$) met criteria for current PTSD but did not meet criteria for lifetime polysubstance dependence (PTSD-SUD). Those respondents with current PTSD and with or without lifetime polysubstance dependence did not differ by age (χ^2 (1, $N = 69$) = .00, $p = .98$), education level (χ^2 (1, $N = 69$) = 1.14, $p = .29$), marital status (χ^2 (2, $N = 69$) = 4.19, $p = .12$), and whether the respondent had minor children (χ^2 (1, $N = 41$) = 1.08, $p = .30$). The two groups differed on minority status (χ^2 (1, $N = 69$) = 5.65, $p = .03$), with the PTSD-SUD/LPD having fewer ethnic minorities than those with PTSD-SUD (27.3% versus 55.6%, respectively). There were no significant differences between the two groups on number of previous sentences (χ^2 (1, $N = 69$) = .02, $p = .90$), whether the crime was a misdemeanor or felony (χ^2 (1, $N = 69$) = .62, $p = .43$), or the length of sentence (χ^2 (1, $N = 41$) = .87, $p = .35$).

A series of independent samples t-tests were conducted to examine differences between the two groups on trauma history, trauma-related symptomatology, and other clinical variables (see Table 2). Significant differences between the two groups were found on the number of total traumatic events overall, $t(67) = -2.66$, $p = .01$, $d = .64$. There were also differences between the two groups on trauma exposure, specifically related to general disasters, $t(67) = -2.03$, $p = .04$, $d = .50$, and crime-related events, $t(67) = -2.35$, $p = .02$, $d = .55$. No differences were found between the groups for experiences of physical/sexual trauma, $t(67) = -1.53$, $p = .13$, $d = .37$. Those women with PTSD-SUD/LPD reported significantly more exposure to trauma with medium to large effects, when compared to PTSD-SUD women.

Comparisons between the two groups on trauma-related symptomatology yielded marginal effects for dissociation, $t(67) = -1.65$, $p = .10$, $d = .40$, anxiety, $t(67) = -1.84$, $p = .07$, $d = .46$, and sexual problems,

TABLE 2. Comparisons Among Incarcerated Women with PTSD and with or Without Lifetime Polysubstance Dependence

Scale	Total		PTSD-No LPS		PTSD-LPS		df	t
	M	SD	M	SD	M	SD		
Trauma History Questionnaire (Total)	11.90	4.00	10.72	3.88	13.18	3.78	67	−2.66**
General	5.25	2.38	4.69	2.34	5.85	2.31	67	−2.03**
Crime	2.01	1.22	1.69	1.19	2.36	1.17	67	−2.35**
Sexual/Physical	4.64	1.75	4.33	1.69	4.97	1.78	67	−1.53
Trauma Symptom Checklist (Total)	1.34	0.59	1.24	0.59	1.46	0.58	67	−1.51
Dissociation	1.39	0.68	1.26	0.67	1.53	0.67	67	−1.65*
Anxiety	1.22	0.64	1.08	0.62	1.36	0.65	67	−1.84*
Depression	1.45	0.61	1.39	0.65	1.51	0.56	67	−0.81
Sexual abuse	1.32	0.67	1.20	0.66	1.45	0.68	67	−1.57
Sleep disturbance	1.93	0.86	1.91	0.87	1.95	0.86	67	−0.20
Sexual problems	0.92	0.70	0.77	0.63	1.08	0.75	67	−1.81*
Addiction Severity Index								
Alcohol	0.36	0.32	0.28	0.30	0.44	0.33	67	−2.11**
Drug	0.30	0.16	0.23	0.14	0.37	0.15	67	−3.91**
Medical	0.41	0.42	0.45	0.44	0.36	0.40	67	0.86
Employment	0.92	0.15	0.97	0.08	0.87	0.18	67	3.07**
Family	0.75	0.91	0.81	0.92	0.70	0.92	67	0.49
Legal	0.40	0.24	0.36	0.26	0.45	0.20	61	−1.54
Psychiatric	0.63	0.19	0.61	0.17	0.65	0.22	61	−0.69

Note. PTSD = posttraumatic stress disorder; LPS = lifetime polysubstance dependence.
* $p \leq .10$, ** $p < .05$.

$t(67) = -1.81, p = .07, d = .44$. Those PTSD-SUD/LPD women reported more trauma-related symptomatology in a number of different domains with small to medium effects, when compared to PTSD-SUD women. Additional questions related to the presence of guilt and dissociation symptoms found in the CAPs indicated that PTSD-SUD/LPD respondents were more likely to experience survivor guilt (24.2% versus 2.8%), $\chi^2 (1, N = 69) = 6.69, p = .01, \phi = .32$, and derealization (23.3% versus 5.9%), $\chi^2 (1, N = 64) = 4.02, p = .04, \phi = .25$, than PTSD-SUD respondents. There were no differences between the two groups on guilt,

$\chi^2(1, N = 68) = 2.94, p = .09, \phi = .21$, depersonalization, $\chi^2(1, N = 64) = 1.90, p = .17, \phi = .17$, or a reduction of awareness, $\chi^2(1, N = 64) = .64, p = .42, \phi = .10$.

In terms of severity of substance use, comparisons indicate expected differences between the two groups in degree of alcohol use, $t(67) = -2.11, p = .04, d = .51$, and drug use, $t(67) = -3.91, p = .00, d = .94$, demonstrating that PTSD-SUD/LPD respondents reported more alcohol and drug severity with medium to large effects, when compared to those who meet the criteria for PTSD-SUD exclusively. The only other ASI subscale that was significantly different between the two groups was employment, $t(67) = 3.07, p = .00, d = -.78$, indicating that those with PTSD-SUD report more impairment with a large effect, when compared to those with PTSD-SUD/LPD.

DISCUSSION

In a sample of incarcerated women with current PTSD and SUD one month prior to incarceration, the current study found that approximately half also met criteria for lifetime polysubstance dependence. Incarcerated women with lifetime polysubstance use, when compared to women without lifetime polysubstance dependence, reported experiencing more traumatic events overall, including specific types of traumatic events specifically crime-related events and general disasters. Trends indicated that those with polysubstance dependence also had higher levels of trauma-related symptomatology related to dissociation, anxiety, and sexual problems than those without polysubstance dependence. On measures of PTSD-related symptomatology, those with polysubstance dependence had a higher prevalence of specific types of guilt (i.e., survivor guilt) and dissociation (i.e., derealization), when compared to those without polysubstance dependence. Finally, incarcerated women with polysubstance dependence reported greater severity of alcohol and drug use when compared to those individuals without lifetime polysubstance dependence. No significant differences were found between the two groups on the number of sexual or physical traumatic events experienced, other PTSD-related symptoms (i.e., general feelings of guilt, dissociation-related areas such as depersonalization, lack of awareness regarding one's surroundings), or other functional impairments (i.e., medical, legal, family/social, psychiatric).

Contrary to expectation, women without polysubstance dependence reported more functional impairment related to employment when compared to those with polysubstance dependence, although this is most likely related to the high rates of unemployment overall (63.6%), as well as the high rates of unemployment among women without polysubstance dependence when compared to those in the polysubstance dependence group (71.9% and 69.0%, respectively). Additional research is needed to further examine the extent to which polysubstance dependence is related to increased impairment in a number of functional areas among populations with co-occuring PTSD and SUD.

Our findings suggest that polysubstance dependence affects many incarcerated women with co-occurring PTSD and SUD. The current study, combined with supportive empirical literature related to polysubstance dependence and trauma exposure with other populations, suggest that women with comorbid PTSD-SUD and lifetime polysubstance dependence may have different experiences, and therefore potentially different treatment needs, than those with PTSD and single substance dependence. Specifically, the current study suggests that this comorbid group of women may have a worse clinical profile in specific areas, especially in the severity of their alcohol and drug use one month prior to incarceration and some of the associated features of PTSD (e.g., derealization, survivor's guilt). Given these differences, women with comorbid polysubstance dependence may benefit from exclusively tailored interventions.

Previous research with other populations (e.g., veterans, individuals who are homeless) has also suggested that polysubstance dependence is associated with more deleterious physical and psychological outcomes for those individuals than for those with a single substance dependence (Agosti & Levin, 2006; Booth, Sullivan, Koegel, & Burnam, 2002; Cottler et al., 2001; Tomasson & Vaglum, 1998; Triffleman, Marmar, Delucchi, & Ronfeldt, 1995). The current study is consistent with previous findings and contributes to extant literature by noting differences between incarcerated women with comorbid PTSD and SUD with and without polysubstance dependence on trauma characteristics (e.g., number of traumas, type of trauma), trauma-related symptoms (e.g., dissociation, anxiety), severity of alcohol and drug use, and psychosocial functioning (e.g., legal problems, psychiatric difficulties, employment status). Specifically, incarcerated women with comorbid PTSD and SUD with polysubstance dependence reported significantly more dysfunction than those without polysubstance dependence.

Substance abuse itself can be seen as a dissociative response to trauma because it disrupts the integration of conscious thought, allowing for the avoidance of aversive memories (Miranda, Meyerson, Long, Marx, & Simpson, 2002). Path analyses examining this "self-medication hypothesis" (Khantzian, 1985) have found evidence that substance use does provide negative reinforcement against the myriad of emotional consequences accompanying the experience of trauma (Miranda et al., 2002; Polusny & Follette, 1995). The self medication hypothesis also purports that PTSD symptoms may play a causal role in substance dependence, which in turn could pose an additional risk to substance dependent individuals such that these individuals are in more situations in which crime-related events are likely to occur. While no studies have specifically attempted to examine this hypothesis among incarcerated women, one longitudinal study with veterans reported that, after controlling for prior drug use, those experiencing PTSD symptoms at 18-24 months reported increased drug use up to 6 years later (Shipherd, Stafford, & Tanner, 2005). While women with co-occurring PTSD and SUD and polysubstance dependence report greater exposure to general disasters and crime-related trauma, it is unclear whether the increased substance use reported among these women may also place these individuals at increased risk for specific types of traumatic events (e.g., crime-related violence). Additional research is needed to establish causal links between trauma exposure, PTSD, and polysubstance dependence among this population.

Future research is also needed to explore the associations between comorbid PTSD and lifetime polysubstance dependence as they relate to trauma exposure (e.g., types of trauma experienced, age of onset) and other PTSD-related symptomatology, including dissociation. It should be noted that although measures of dissociation and guilt were generally high within the sample, the current study did not find differences between women with and without polysubstance dependence in dissociation (e.g., depersonalization) and a more general measure of guilt. The current study did find that women with polysubstance dependence, when compared to those without the polysubstance dependence, were more likely to have symptoms related to guilt and derealization, a type of dissociation. Since women with lifetime polysubstance dependence also reported experiencing more exposure to general disasters and crime-related trauma, it is possible that their greater levels of survivor guilt and derealization were linked to these traumatic experiences. Other researchers have also found that specific types of trauma (e.g., emotional abuse experienced during childhood), while not associated with overall scores of dissociation, were associated with increases in specific dissociative features (e.g., depersonalization; Briere, 2006;

Simeon, Guralnik, Schmeidler, Sirof, & Knutelska, 2001). Based on these results, future research may benefit from examining whether different traumatic experiences are etiologically linked to subtypes of dissociative responses.

Limitations to the present study warrant additional attention. Given the lack of previous literature comparing incarcerated women with PTSD and comorbid polysubstance dependence to those with PTSD-SUD, the decision was made to discuss findings showing marginal significance (p<.10), although this decision increases the likelihood of error. Additionally, previous research has suggested that retrospective reports of physical and sexual-related trauma may result in an underreporting of early trauma, indicating a potential underestimation in the experience of trauma for these women (Williams, 1994). The current study may have been additionally enhanced by a larger sample size and the inclusion of those without polysubstance dependence, substance use disorder, or PTSD. Lastly, larger sample, longitudinal studies with the ability to examine individual trajectories of PTSD and substance use could potentially shed light on more complex relationships with substance use and dependence, particularly for incarcerated women, but also for broader community samples.

Despite such limitations, attaining additional knowledge about the experiences of those with comorbid polysubstance dependence and PTSD can give clinicians information about designing treatments for this at-risk group. This is particularly essential for prison-based samples, because for women exposed to previous trauma, prison could potentially offer "an environment of relative physical and psychological safety . . . (and) may be an effective time for a woman to address the effects of prior victimization" (Bradley & Davino, 2002, p. 352).

REFERENCES

Agosti, V., & Levin, F. R. (2006). The effects of alcohol and drug dependence on the course of depression. *American Journal of Addiction, 15*, 71-75.

American Correctional Association. (1991). *The female offender: What will the future hold?* Arlington, VA: Kirby Lithographic Company.

Blake, D. D., Weathers, F. W., Nagy, L. M., Kaloupek, D. G., Klauminzer, G., Charney, D., et al. (1990). A clinical rating scale for assessing current and lifetime PTSD: The CAPS- 1. *Behavior Therapy, 18*, 187-188.

Booth, B. M., Sullivan, G., Koegel, P., & Burnam, A. (2002). Vulnerability factors for homelessness associated with substance dependence in a community sample of homeless adults. *American Journal of Drug and Alcohol Use, 28*(3), 429-452.

Brady, K. T., Killeen, T., Saladin, M. E., Dansky, B. S., & Becker, S. (1994). Comorbid substance abuse and posttraumatic stress disorder: Characteristics of women in treatment. *American Journal on Addictions, 3*, 160-164.

Bradley, R. G., & Davino, K. M. (2002). Perceptions of the prison environment: When prison is "the safest place I've ever been." *Psychology of Women Quarterly, 26*, 351-359.

Briere, J., & Runtz, M. (1989). The Trauma Symptom Checklist (TSC-33): Early data on a new scale. *Journal of Interpersonal Violence, 4*, 151-163.

Brown, P. J., & Wolfe, J. (1994). Substance abuse and posttraumatic stress disorder comorbidity. *Drug and Alcohol Dependence, 35*, 51-59.

Browne, A., Miller, B., & Maguin, E. (1999). Prevalence and severity of lifetime physical and sexual victimization among incarcerated women. *International Journal of Law and Psychiatry, 22*(3-4), 301-322.

Cook, S. L., Smith, S. G., Tusher, C. P., & Raiford, J. (2005). Self-reports of traumatic events in a random sample of incarcerated women. *Women & Criminal Justice, 16*, 107-126.

Cottler, L. B., Compton, W. M., Mager, D., Spitznagel, E. L., & Janca, A. (1992). Posttraumatic stress disorder among substance users from the general population. *American Journal of Psychiatry, 149*, 664-670.

Cottler, L. B., Nishith, P., & Compton, W. M. III (2001). Gender differences in risk factors for trauma exposure and post-traumatic stress disorder among inner-city drug abusers in and out of treatment. *Comprehensive Psychiatry, 42*, 111-117.

Covington, S. (1998). Women in prison: Approaches in the treatment of our most invisible population. In J. Harden & M. Hill (Eds.), *Breaking the rules: Women in prison and feminist therapy* (pp.141-153). New York: The Haworth Press, Inc.

Dansky, B. S., Roitzsch, J. C., Brady, K. T. & Saladin, M. E. (1997). Posttraumatic stress disorder and substance abuse: Use of research in a clinical setting. *Journal of Traumatic Stress, 10*, 141-148.

Desjardins, L., Brochu, S., & Biron, L. L. (1992). *Etude epidemiologique slur la consommation de psychotropes chez les contrevenantes incarcerees. Rapport de recherche.* (Epidemiological study on the use of drugs within a population of incarcerated women. Research report.) Montreal: Universite de Montreal. C.I.C.C.

Druley, K. A., & Pashko, S. (1988). Post-Traumatic Stress Disorder in Word War II and Korean combat veterans with alcohol dependence. In M. Galanter (Ed.), *Recent development in alcoholism* (Vol. 6, pp. 89-101). New York: Plenum Press.

First, M. B., Spitzer, R. L., Gibbon, M., & Williams, J. B. W. (1997). *Structured clinical interview for DSM-IV Axis I Disorders: Clinician version: Administration booklet.* Washington, DC: American Psychiatric Press.

Goldenberg, I. M., Mueller, T., Fierman, E. J., Gordon, A., Pratt, L., Cox, K., Park, T., Lavori, P., Goisman, R. M., & Keller, M. B. (1995). Specificity of substance abuse in anxiety disordered subjects. *Comprehensive Psychiatry, 36*, 31 9-328.

Greene, B. L. (1996). Trauma History Questionnaire. In B. H. Stamm (Ed.), *Measurement of stress, trauma, and adaptation* (pp. 366-369). Lutherville, MD: Sidran Press.

Helzer J. E., Robins L. N., & McEvoy L. (1987). Post-traumatic stress disorder in the general population. Findings of the epidemiologic catchment area survey. *New England Journal of Medicine, 317,* 1630-1634.

Jordan, B. K., Schlenger, W. E., Fairbank, J. A., & Caddell, J. M. (1996). Prevalence of psychiatric disorders among incarcerated women. II: Convicted felons entering prison. *Archives of General Psychiatry, 53,* 513-519.

Kessler, R. C., Sonnega, A., Bromet, E. J., Hughes, M., & Nelson, C. B. (1995). Posttraumatic National Comorbidity Survey. *Archives of General Psychiatry, 52,* 1048-1060.

Khantzian, E. J. (1985). The self-medication hypothesis of addictive disorders: Focus on heroin and cocaine dependence. *American Journal of Psychiatry, 142,* 1259-1264.

Kilpatrick, D., Resnick, H., Saunders, B., & Best, C. (1996). *Victimization, post-traumatic stress disorder, and substance use abuse among women.* Drug Addiction Research and Health of Women (NIH Publication No. 98-4290, pp, 285-307). Rockville, MD: US Department of Health and Human Services.

Kubiak, S. P. (2004). The effects of PTSD on treatment adherence, drug relapse, and criminal recidivism in a sample of incarcerated men and women. *Research on Social Work Practice,* 424-433.

Kulka, R. A., Schlenger, W. E., Fairbank, J. A., Hough, R. L., Jordan, B. K., Marmar, C. R., & Weiss, D. S. (1990). Trauma and the Vietnam War generation: Report of findings from the National Vietnam Veterans Readjustment Study. New York: BrunnedMazel. Abstracted in *PTSD Research Quarterly, 1*(3), 4-5.

Lake, E. S. (1993). An exploration of the violent victim experiences of female offenders. *Violence and Victims, 8,* 41-51.

Lewis, C. F. (2005a). Post-Traumatic Stress Disorder in HIV-positive incarcerated women. *Journal of the American Academy of Psychiatry and the Law, 33,* 455-464.

Lewis, C. F. (2005b). Female offenders in correctional settings. In C. L. Scott and J. B. Gerbasi (Eds.) *Handbook of Correctional Mental Health.* (pp. 155-185). Arlington, VA: American Psychiatric Publishing, Inc.

Maeve, M. K. (2000). Speaking unavoidable truths: Understanding early childhood sexual and physical violence among women in prison. *Issues in Mental Health Nursing, 21,* 473-498.

McGahan, P. L., Griffith, J. A., Parente, R., & McLellan, A. T. (1986). *Addiction Severity Index: Composite scores manual.* Philadelphia: Treatment Research Institute.

McLellan, A. T., Kushner, H., Metzger, D., Peters, R., et al. (1992). The fifth edition of the Addiction Severity Index. *Journal of Substance Abuse Treatment, 9*(3), 199-213.

Miranda, R., Meverson, L. A., Long, P. J., Marx, B. P., & Simpson, S. M. (2002). Sexual assault and alcohol use: Exploring the self-medication hypothesis. *Violence and Victims, 17,* 205-217.

Najavits, L. M. (2002). *Seeking Safety: A treatment manual for PTSD and substance abuse.* New York, NY: Guilford.

Najavits, L. M., Weiss, R. D., & Shaw, S. R. (1997). The link between substance abuse and PTSD in women: A research review. *American Journal of Addictions, 6,* 273-283.

Najavits, L. M., Weiss, R. D., Shaw, S. R., & Muenz, L. R. (1998). Seeking Safety: Outcome of a new cognitive-behavioral psychotherapy for women with post-traumatic stress disorder and substance dependence. *Journal of Traumatic Stress, 11*, 437-456.

Ouimette, P. C., Wolfe, J., & Chrestman, K. R. (1996). Characteristics of Posttraumatic Stress Disorder-alcohol abuse comorbidity in women. *Journal of Substance Abuse, 8*, 335-346.

Ouimette, P. C., Ahrens, C., Moos, R. H., & Finney, J. W. (1997). Posttraumatic stress disorder in substance abuse patients: Relationship to one-year posttreatment outcomes. *Psychology of Addictive Behavior, 11*, 34-47.

Parsons, M. L., & Warner-Robbins, C. (2002). Factors that support women's successful transition to the community following jail/prison. *Health Care for Women International, 23*(1), 6-18.

Peters, R. H., Greenbaum, P. E., Edens, J. F., Carter, C. R., & Ortiz, M. M. (1998). Prevalence of DSM-IV substance abuse and dependence disorders among prison inmates. *American Journal of Drug and Alcohol Abuse, 24*, 573-87.

Polusny, M. A., & Follette, V. M. (1995). Long-term correlates of child sexual abuse: Theory and review of empirical literature. *Applied and Preventive Psychology, 4*, 148-166.

Resnick, H. S., Kilpatrick, D. G., Dansky, B. S., Saunders, B. E. & Best, C. L. (1993). Prevalence of trauma and Posttraumatic Stress Disorder in a representative national sample of women. *Journal of Consulting and Clinical Psychology, 61*, 984-991.

Richie, B. E. (2001). Challenges incarcerated women face as they return to their communities: Findings from life history interviews. *Crime and Delinquency, 47*(3), 368-389.

Shipherd, J. C., Stafford, J., & Tanner, L. R. (2005). Predicting alcohol and drug abuse in Persian Gulf War veterans: What role do PTSD symptoms play? *Addictive Behaviors, 30*, 595-599.

Simeon, D., Guralnik, O., Schmeidler, J., Sirof, B., & Knutelska, M. (2001). The role of childhood interpersonal trauma in Depersonalization Disorder. *American Journal of Psychiatry, 158*, 1027-1033.

Singer, M. I., Bussey, J., Song, L.-Y., & Lunghofer, L. (1995). The psychosocial issues of women serving time in jail. *Social Work, 40*(1), 103-113.

Teplin, L. A., Abram, K. M., & McClelland, G. M. (1 996). Prevalence of psychiatric disorders among incarcerated women, I: Pretrial jail detainees. *Archives of General Psychiatry, 53*, 505-512.

Tomasson, K., & Vaglum, P. (1998). The role of psychiatric comorbidity in the prediction of readmission for detoxification. *Comprehensive Psychiatry, 39*, 129-136.

Triffleman, E. G., Marmar, C. R., Delucchi, K. L., & Ronfeldt, H. (1995). Childhood trauma and posttraumatic stress disorder in substance abuse inpatients. *Journal of Nervous and Mental Disease, 183*, 172-176.

U. S. Department of Justice. (1999). *Women offenders* (Special Report, NCJ 175688). Washington, DC: Bureau of Justice Statistics.

Weathers, F. W., Ruscio, A. M., & Keane, T. M. (1999). Psychometric properties of nine scoring rules for the Clinician-Administered Posttraumatic Stress Disorder Scale. *Psychological Assessment, 11*, 124-133.

Weitzel, S. L., & Blount, W. R. (1982). Incarcerated female felons and substance abuse. *Journal of Drug Issues, 12,* 259-273.

Williams, L. M. (1994). Recall of childhood trauma: A prospective study of women's memories of child sexual abuse. *Journal of Consulting and Clinical Psychology, 62,* 1167-1176.

Zlotnick, C. (1997). Posttraumatic Stress Disorder (PTSD), PTSD comorbidity, and childhood abuse among incarcerated women. *The Journal of Nervous and Mental Disease, 185,* 761-763.

Zlotnick, C. (2002). *Treatment of Incarcerated Women with Substance Abuse and Posttraumatic Stress Disorder, Final Report (#195165).* Rockville, MD, National Criminal Justice Reference Service (NCJRS).

Zlotnick, C., Bruce, S. E., Weisberg, R. B., Shea, T., Machan, J. T., & Kelling, M. B. (2003a). Social and health functioning in female primary care patients with Posttraumatic Stress Disorder with or without comorbid substance abuse. *Comprehensive Psychiatry, 44,* 177-183.

Zlotnick, C., Najavits, L. M., Rohsevow, D. J., & Johnson, D. (2003b). A cognitive-behavioral treatment for incarcerated women with Substance Abuse Disorder and Posttraumatic Stress Disorder: Findings from a pilot study. *Journal of Substance Abuse Treatment, 25,* 99-105.

doi:10.1300/J229v08n02_02

Levels of Trauma Among Women Inmates with HIV Risk and Alcohol Use Disorders: Behavioral and Emotional Impacts

Megan R. Hebert, MA
Jennifer S. Rose, PhD
Cynthia Rosengard, PhD, MPH
Jennifer G. Clarke, MD, MPH
Michael D. Stein, MD

SUMMARY. An increasing number of women are involved in the criminal justice system. Women in corrections are often of low socio-economic status, medically underserved and exposed to a variety of traumatic events. Programs and services provided in correctional settings

Megan R. Hebert is affiliated with Rhode Island Hospital Substance Abuse Research Unit, DGIM, Providence, RI.

Jennifer S. Rose is affiliated with Brown University Medical School, Providence, RI and Rhode Island Hospital Substance Abuse Research Unit, DGIM, Providence, RI.

Cynthia Rosengard is affiliated with Brown University Medical School, Providence, RI and Rhode Island Hospital Substance Abuse Research Unit, DGIM, Providence, RI.

Jennifer G. Clarke is affiliated with Brown University Medical School, Providence, RI and Memorial Hospital of Rhode Island, Pawtucket, RI.

Michael D. Stein is affiliated with Brown University Medical School, Providence, RI and Rhode Island Hospital Substance Abuse Research Unit, DGIM, Providence, RI.

Address correspondence to: Michael D. Stein, Rhode Island Hospital, DGIM Research, 593 Eddy Street (Plain Building), Providence, RI 02903 (E-mail: mstein@lifespan.org).

[Haworth co-indexing entry note]: "Levels of Trauma Among Women Inmates with HIV Risk and Alcohol Use Disorders: Behavioral and Emotional Impacts." Hebert, Megan R. et al. Co-published simultaneously in *Journal of Trauma & Dissociation* (The Haworth Medical Press, an imprint of The Haworth Press, Inc.) Vol. 8, No. 2, 2007, pp. 27-46; and: *Trauma and Dissociation in Convicted Offenders: Gender, Science, and Treatment Issues* (ed: Kathryn Quina, and Laura S. Brown) The Haworth Medical Press, an imprint of The Haworth Press, Inc., 2007, pp. 27-46. Single or multiple copies of this article are available for a fee from The Haworth Document Delivery Service [1-800-HAWORTH, 9:00 a.m. - 5:00 p.m. (EST). E-mail address: docdelivery@haworthpress.com].

should be informed by the unique profiles and needs of these women. This study sought to identify distinct sub-groups (classes) of incarcerated women based on differences in their qualitative (types of trauma) and quantitative (number of) trauma experiences. Demographics, psychosocial and behavioral characteristics were measured in 149 women entering jail, who reported recent hazardous drinking and HIV sexual risk behavior. Two classes based on trauma exposure of women were identified through latent class analysis. The classes did not differ with respect to qualitative differences in trauma exposure (both classes reported all forms of trauma), but did differ with respect to quantitative differences (Class 2 reported more exposure to trauma in all categories than Class 1). The classes also differed significantly on current psychological functioning, alcohol treatment, problems, and consequences, drug histories, sexual risk, medical conditions, and social group characteristics. In all areas, members of Class 2 were significantly more likely to report higher levels of measured variables. Nearly all women in our sample reported levels of trauma exposure, suggesting a need for intervention and attention. Through identifying these separate classes, limited resources for trauma survivors in the correctional setting could be most appropriately allocated. doi:10.1300/J229v08n02_03 *[Article copies available for a fee from The Haworth Document Delivery Service: 1-800-HAWORTH. E-mail address: <docdelivery@haworthpress.com> Website: <http://www.HaworthPress.com>* © 2007 by The Haworth Press, Inc. All rights reserved.]

KEYWORDS. Women inmates, trauma exposure, risk behaviors

INTRODUCTION

Studies commonly find that women inmates have higher rates of health problems than men inmates or women in the general population. Incarcerated women have an HIV prevalence of 3.5% compared with 2.2% for incarcerated men (Greenfeld & Snell, 1999). Incarcerated women are also three times more likely to report their health is poor (Marquart, Brewer, Mullings, and Crouch, 1999) compared to women in the general population. The prevalence of substance abuse among incarcerated women is greater than 60 percent and felony convictions for drug possession increased 41% among women between 1990 and 1996. Furthermore, between 7-24% of female inmates were using alcohol, 11-32% were using drugs, and 10-18% were using both at the time they committed their offense (Greenfield & Snell, 1999). Seventy percent of female arrestees, more than twice the amount of male arrestees, have lifetime prevalence rates of alcohol abuse or dependence (Levin, Blanch, & Jennings, 1998).

These disproportionate rates of health problems place an enormous burden on correctional facilities, both in terms of cost and need to provide medications and treatment regimens. In addition, for many women, addictive behaviors are the direct or indirect cause of their incarceration, with the majority of women found guilty of drug use or nonviolent crimes committed for money to purchase drugs. At the same time, problem behaviors such as sexual risk and substance use may be modifiable, if we commit resources appropriately while women are in prison. Thus, understanding the precursors of these behaviors could guide appropriate interventions to help reduce the level of problem behaviors once a woman is released, thus reducing the likelihood of reincarceration.

The demands of addressing mental health needs can be as great as those of physical health needs. Several studies have shown that rates of PTSD are substantially higher among detained women (Green, Miranda, Doaroowalla, & Siddique, 2005; Teplin, Abram, & McClelland, 1996; Zlotnick, 1997). Although an important component of addressing this population's mental health needs, the high prevalence of PTSD remains largely unexamined, including the potential for dissociative problems in functioning within the prison system.

Few studies have examined the prevalence and effects of a range of traumatic events among incarcerated women on their presenting risk behaviors. Similar to the limited national studies conducted to date, those involving incarcerated women generally fail to focus on trauma. If examined at all, trauma is often a secondary outcome, or when it is of primary importance, is limited to a particular type (i.e., sexual) and/or occurs within the context of a treatment-seeking sample (Bradley & Follingstad, 2003; Sanders & McNeill, 1997). The narrow research that has been conducted nonetheless provides unquestionable evidence that trauma, particularly interpersonal, is highly prevalent among female inmates. The only study to have assessed a range of trauma exposures, as a primary focus, within a sample of incarcerated women found that 98% had experienced at least one type of trauma (Green et al., 2005). However, there remains an important need to examine specific dynamics (e.g., underlying classes) of additional associated risks (e.g., drug use, sex risk behavior, social group characteristics) as they relate to incarcerated women's past trauma experiences.

Findings from a national random sample of 3,362 adults showed that those who reported childhood sexual abuse as occurring prior to puberty were significantly more likely to be incarcerated both in later adolescence and as adults (Curtis, Leung, Sullivan, Eschbach, & Stinson, 2001). Examination of the rates and effects of trauma among this population have revealed that incarcerated women have significantly high rates of physical and/or sexual abuse histories, ranging from 40-80% (Austin, Bloom, & Donahue, 1992; Brennan & Austin, 1997; Browne, Miller, & Maguin, 1999; Greenfeld & Snell, 1999; Harlow, 1999). Browne, Miller, and Maguin (1999) found that not only was the prevalence of abuse much higher among incarcerated women than in the general population, but also that the frequency and severity of abuse is greater.

Girls who experienced childhood sexual abuse, compared to those who had experienced other types of victimization and those who had no histories of victimization, are at a higher risk of being involved in and/or arrested for prostitution as adults (Mullings, Marquart, & Brewer, 2000; Paone & Chavkin, 1993; Widom & Ames, 1994). Similarly, Widom (1995) found that compared to controls and victims of childhood physical abuse and neglect, childhood sexual abuse survivors differed on likelihood of arrest for prostitution and were 27.7 times more likely to be arrested for this crime than the control group. Trauma exposure is associated with significantly higher rates of substance use (Hill, Blow, Young, & Singer, 1994; McNutt, Carlson, Persaud, & Postmus, 2002). In the general population, Felitti et al. (1998) found a dose-response relationship between the count of traumatic exposures and various outcomes including depression, illicit drug use, and alcoholism. Other research demonstrates that outcomes such as adult sexual assault, physical health, and crime involvement are associated with particular types of trauma but not with other types of trauma (e.g., childhood sexual abuse, but not childhood physical abuse as a predictor of adult sexual assault and physical assault by a commercial sex partner as a predictor of incarceration during the last year but not sexual assault) nor associated with no trauma exposure (El-Bassel et al., 2001; Gil-Rivas, Fiorentine, Anglin & Taylor, 1997; Messerman-Moore & Brown, 2004; Mullings et al., 2000; Widom, 1995).

While trauma is essential to a diagnosis of PTSD, again, the links between problem behaviors and PTSD have been largely ignored in both health psychology and corrections. Alcohol and substance misuse are common in women exposed to trauma and PTSD has been theorized to mediate this relationship, as alcohol and drugs are oftentimes used to cope with the PTSD symptoms (Epstein, Saunders, Kilpatrick, & Resnick, 1998). The DSM-IV PTSD field trials indicate that early onset and prolonged exposure to trauma, common among women inmates, are predictors of what has been theorized as complex PTSD or disorders of extreme stress (DES). Characterized by more severe and additional symptoms than PTSD, the field trials found that these individuals had more symptoms of affect regulation, dissociation, and somatization. This is of particular importance as the manifestations of these symptoms such as anger modulation, self-destructiveness, suicidal behavior, excessive risk taking, sexual involvement, chronic pain, and interpersonal relationship problems are prevalent among incarcerated women (Roth, Newman, Pelcovitz, van der Kolk, & Mandel, 1997).

The purpose of this study was to explore whether there exist distinct subgroups (classes) of women inmates based on patterns of trauma. It is proposed that different types and number of trauma exposures will result in distinct classes characterized by, and differing significantly in, risk behaviors and psychosocial profiles.

Specifically, it is hypothesized that among these women, we will identify classes that are both qualitatively distinct in terms of the types of trauma experienced and quantitatively distinct in terms of the number of trauma exposures experienced. Periods of incarceration provide unique public health opportunities to offer needed services to an underserved population. By identifying subgroups of women, interventions and limited service resources can be more beneficially directed.

METHOD

Sample

Participants were the first 149 women enrolled in an ongoing randomized clinical trial assessing the effects of a brief motivationally based intervention on post-release drinking and sexual risk behaviors of women who report hazardous drinking and engaging in HIV risk behaviors prior to their incarceration. Women were recruited for this longitudinal study as they entered the Women's Facility of the Rhode Island Department of Corrections (RI DOC). The RI DOC is a cohesive correctional system holding all levels of inmates including those awaiting arraignment or trial and those who are sentenced.

Study approval was obtained from the Miriam Hospital Institutional Review Board, the Office for Human Research Protection and the Medical Research Advisory Group at the ACI before starting the study. A Certificate of Confidentiality was obtained from the federal government to further ensure participant privacy. The warden of the women's facility agreed to help guarantee participant confidentiality and granted permission for all interactions with the women to occur one-on-one with trained, female research assistants in unmonitored rooms.

After detained women had completed the facility intake process, research assistants (RAs) attempted to screen all women for the clinical trial. Screening was done confidentially and with verbal consent. Each morning RAs recorded all new commitments from the traffic sheets into a log that was kept continuously throughout the study period. The RA would construct a list of all available inmates who had not yet been contacted during that commitment. The list would then be given to an assigned correctional officer who would coordinate with officers on the cell wings to have the inmates sent individually to the private room used to conduct screens. Although the warden was aware of the study content, specific research objectives were not shared with the officers so as not to jeopardize participant confidentiality. Officers were told only that the questionnaire was for a research study and that all women committed to the ACI were eligible for potential participation.

The primary aims of the randomized clinical trial are to test the hypotheses that among this population of women who have engaged in hazardous drinking and HIV-risk behaviors and are returning to the community, a brief alcohol intervention will result in less alcohol use at follow-up compared to standard of care and that drinking will mediate the effect of the brief intervention on HIV-risk taking outcomes. Thus, eligibility criteria included: plans to reside in Rhode Island for a period of 6 months following release (for follow-up purposes), English speaking, recent levels of hazardous drinking (≥ 4 drinks on one occasion 3 or more times in the 90 days prior to incarceration, or ≥ 8 drinks per week on average in the 90 prior to incarceration, or $\geq$ a score of 8 on the Alcohol Use Identification Disorders Test), and recent engagement in an HIV risk behavior (engaging in unprotected male-female vaginal sex ≥ 3 times in the 90 days prior to incarceration or sharing injection drug equipment ≥ 3 times in the 90 days prior to incarceration).

Following screening, a detailed written informed consent was read aloud to each eligible woman who wished to participate. It was emphasized that study participation was completely voluntary and would not affect status or services received in the facility or community. In total, 1,308 women were screened throughout a 25-month period, of which 1,029 did not meet the primary inclusion criteria of recent HIV risk and/ or hazardous levels of drinking. An additional 132 women were not eligible due to residence location, language barriers, or lack of consent comprehension. Forty-one women were eligible but did not want to participate, yielding a participation rate of 78% (149/190).

The data used in this analysis were extrapolated from the baseline interview, which was conducted in the RI DOC and lasted an average of 45 to 60 minutes. Every participant was compensated $20 in the form of a money order, which was mailed to her the day after her release. If a participant was later sentenced, she was given the option to have it deposited into her RI DOC account.

Analyses

Classes of women inmates were identified first using latent class analysis (LCA; McCutcheon, 1987). LCA is a type of cluster analysis in which the specific number of groups and their characteristics are not known. Two particular advantages of using LCA over standard cluster analysis are that observed variables do not need to be scaled and can have different measurement levels and LCA provides a probability statistic of a person belonging to a given class. In forming the classes, LCA assumes that a heterogeneous population of individuals can be grouped into a finite number of homogenous subgroups or classes, with small differences within the groups and large differences between them. We hypothesized that within the sample of women inmates who have hazardous drinking levels and who are engaging in HIV-risk behaviors, a population known to have high exposure to traumas throughout their lifetime, there is a single underlying latent variable that divides the sample into distinct classes.

This analysis tested a set of 3 models specifying one to three classes. The number of final classes to retain is based on the combination of model parsimony, fit statistics, and how theoretically meaningful and different the classes are. Model parsimony was addressed by the use of a likelihood ratio, approximately distributed as a chi-square statistic, and by an evaluation of the Bayes Information Criterion (BIC; Schwarz, 1978) and the Akaike Information Criterion (AIC; Akaike, 1981). A significant chi-square statistic is evidence to reject the model with one less class and when comparing models, smaller values of the BIC and the AIC indicate better fitting ones. Other statistics used to evaluate how many classes to obtain are entropy and class probability. Entropy is an average probability indication based on the number of observations and the number of classes. A perfect value of 1.0 would mean that every individual in all classes has a 100% chance of being put into the class they were assigned. Lower values indicate that classes may not be distinct. Higher values of both entropy and class probability are preferred.

Similar to standard cluster analytic techniques, validation of the latent classes by variables that were not used in the class formation is essential. These validation analyses allow for the characterization of the classes and provide further evidence that there are meaningful differences between the classes. Validation analyses were conducted using analysis of variance (ANOVA) for continuous variables and chi-square difference tests for dichotomous variables. Variables used included demographics, additional trauma related variables, psychological-functioning variables, alcohol-related and drug-related variables, and sexual behavior variables. Due to the number of analyses being conducted, the critical value for indicating statistical significance was set to be more conservative at a level of $p \leq 0.01$.

Class Identification Measures

The variables utilized to identify the subgroups of incarcerated women included 4 types of trauma, each measured by 2 to 13 items. Items that were endorsed were coded as a "1" and items within types of trauma were summed to produce a count variable indicating trauma type exposures. Items were taken from the Trauma History Questionnaire, which has been previously used in samples of incarcerated women (Green, 1996; Zlotnick, Najavitis, Rohsenow, & Johnson, 2003) and are summarized below.

Crime related trauma. The crime related trauma score was composed of 4 items. Each participant was asked if anyone ever: (1) tried to take something from them by use of force, (2) attempted to or actually robbed them, (3) attempted to or actually broke into their home when they were not there, and (4) attempted to or actually broke into their home when they were there.

General disaster and trauma. The score for general disaster and trauma was constructed from the following 13 items: (1) serious accident, (2) experience of a natural disaster, i.e., tornado, earthquake, flood, etc., (3) experience of a man-made disaster, i.e., fire, building collapse, bank robbery, etc., (4) exposure to health threatening chemicals, (5) situation resulting in serious injury to self, (6) situation in which death or serious injury to self was feared, (7) witnessed someone killed or seriously injured, (8) seen or had to handle dead person(s), (9) had a family member or close friend murdered, (10) had a spouse, partner, or child die, (11) had a life-threatening illness, (12) unexpectedly had someone close die or become seriously injured or ill, and (13) engaged in military combat.

Sexual trauma. The sexual trauma score consisted of two items, one assessing rape (vaginal, anal, or oral) and one assessing private touching of their body or made to touch another's under force or threat.

Physical trauma. Physical trauma was assessed by three items that measured: (1) being attacked with a weapon, (2) being attacked without a weapon with serious injury resulting, and (3) being hurt or beaten by a family member hard enough to cause injury.

Validation Measures

Variables used to better characterize the subgroups and describe the distinct differences between them included general descriptives, several questions regarding rape-specific trauma, 3 measures of psychological functioning, alcohol related variables, drug related variables, indicators of sex risk, medical variables, and several indicators measuring social group.

Descriptives. Descriptives included: age at time of interview and dichotomous items assessing: (1) self-rated measure of general health (poor or fair vs. good or better), (2) if the participant had a high school diploma, (3) had been in foster care as a child, and (4) the participant's race or ethnicity.

Additional trauma items. Additional items relating to trauma included dichotomous items assessing the relationship to their perpetrator(s) as family, friend or acquaintance, sex partner, and/or stranger.

Psychological functioning variables. Psychological functioning was measured through the use of three psychometrically validated scales. *Depression* was assessed by the Beck Depression Inventory II, in which a score of 0-13 indicates minimal depression, 14-19 mild, 20-28 moderate, and 29-63 severe (Beck, Steere, & Brown, 1996). The *Posttraumatic Stress Disorder* (PTSD) and the *Generalized Anxiety Disorder* (GAD) subscales of the Psychiatric Diagnostic Screening Questionnaire (PDSQ) were used to evaluate prevalence of these disorders (Zimmerman & Mattia, 2001a). A score of 5 or more on the PTSD scale and 7 or more on the GAD scale is the recommended cutoff for identifying individuals with a positive screen for the disorder. These cutoff points have been found to result in a sensitivity of 90% in correctly identifying the presence of the disorder (Zimmerman & Mattia, 2001b). These variables were dichotomous and measured positive or negative presence of the disorder on the respective diagnostic screen.

Alcohol-related variables. A single dichotomous item assessed any alcohol-related treatment that included detox, residential care, and/or outpatient treatment in the 90 days prior to incarceration. Continuous alcohol-related variables included scores on the Short Inventory of Problems (SIP-2R) assessed alcohol related problems participants experienced in the 90 days prior to incarceration (Feinn, Tennen, & Kranzler, 2003). The SIP-2R is a 15-item instrument that yields a total score of 0-45 with continuous cutoffs indicative of an increase in alcohol-related problems. For women, 0-10 is considered "Very Low," 15-16 as "Low," 19-22 as "Medium," 26-29 as "High," and 34 and over as "Very High." Fourteen additional "Yes" or "No" items that measured alcohol consequences were also included and assessed such events like ever having been arrested while under the influence of alcohol, ever having an unplanned pregnancy because of drinking, ever lost a job or left school because of drinking, and ever lost custody of children because of drinking. All responses of "Yes" were coded as "1" and summed for a total score ranging from 0-14. A final alcohol related measure included in this analysis was the age at which a participant reported first being drunk.

Drug-related variables. Variables assessing drug use and drug risk included: (1) any use of heroin or opiates (2) any use of cocaine, (3) age at which a participant first injected any type of drugs, (4) any drug injection, (5) any sharing of drug injection equipment, (6) have or had a main sex-partner who injected drugs, (7) having been to a crack house or shooting gallery once or more times per week, (8) been in a detox, residential care setting or outpatient treatment for drug use and (9) having ever been on methadone. With the exception of age of first injection, having a main partner who injected, and having ever been on methadone, all questions referred only to the 90 days prior to incarceration.

Sex-risk variables. Three items were used to assess sex-risk: (1) self-report of having sex for drugs or money in the 90 days prior to incarceration, (2) reporting never using a condom during sex in the 90 days prior to incarceration, and (3) lifetime number of male sex partners. This variable was measured on a 6-point continuous scale with the following response choices: 0 = 0; 1 = 1; 2 = 2-10; 3 = 11-20; 4 = 21-50; 5 = 51-150 and 6 = 151 or more.

Medical variables. Three medical related variables measured (1) number of self-reported conditions that was a sum of the following: asthma, diabetes, liver disease (hepatitis or cirrhosis), hypertension, cancer, past psychiatric hospitalization(s), and previous heart attack or stroke, (2) whether or not the participant had any form of health insurance coverage, and (3) if they had been to a doctor's office or an emergency room in the prior 90 days.

Social group variables. Social group environment was assessed through the use of 4 variables: (1) score on the Tangible Support subscale of the MOS Social Support Survey (Sherbourne & Stewart, 1991) with "0" reflecting no support and "4" reflecting the most, (2) number of HIV+ family members and friends of the participant, (3) proportion of people the participant spends time with who have a drug or alcohol problem, and (4) proportion of people the participant spends time with who encourages their drinking. The last two variables were measured on a continuous scale with the following points: 0 = None; 1 = Some; 2 = Half; 3 = Most; 4 = All.

RESULTS

LCA Results

Model fit indices of the one-, two-, and three-class models suggested that the two-class solution most adequately explained the data (see Table 1). Although the BIC and the AIC were slightly lower for the three-class solution compared to the two (1982.394, 1928.566 vs. 1983.924, 1928.566), entropy decreased by 6% and the individual class probabilities decreased as well. Further evidence supporting the two-class solution was a non-significant p-value when the three-class model was tested, indicating that a one less class model was a better fit. For the two-class solution, the average latent class probabilities for the most likely latent class membership was 0.93 for class 1 and 0.97 for class 2, evidencing good prediction of actual class membership.

Latent Class Profiles and Validation

Seventy-five women were characterized as belonging to Class 1 and seventy-two women as belonging to Class 2 (Table 2). Two participants did not answer some of the class identification variables and were excluded from further analyses, resulting in an effective sample of 147 women. Classes did not differ significantly based on age, race, or education level. Class 2 was significantly more likely to have experienced greater exposures to different traumas across all trauma types measured than Class 1. Additionally, more than a third of the women in Class 2 reported having been raped by a stranger compared to 13.7% of women in Class 1 (p < 0.003). In terms of current psychological functioning, 89% of women in Class 2 met criteria suggestive of GAD and 90% met

TABLE 1. Model Fit for Tests of 1-3 Class Solutions

Number of Classes	Log Likelihood	Number of Parameters	BIC	AIC	Likelihood Ratio Test p-value	Entropy	Probability
1	−1023.591	8	2087.105	2063.182	NA	NA	1.0 1 = .933
2	−959.524	13	1983.924	1945.049	<0.001	.844	2 = .971 1 = .836
3	−946.283	18	1982.394	1928.566	0.1650	.781	2 = .964 3 = .882

TABLE 2. Class Profile on LCA Variables

LCA Variable	Class 1 (n = 75)	Class 2 (n = 72)	p-value
Descriptives			
Age	33.2 (8.5)	35.0 (9.1)	0.209
Self-Rating of Good or Better Health	80.0%	50.0%	<0.001
HS Diploma	32.0%	38.9%	0.383
Foster Care as a Child	18.1%	33.3%	0.037
Race			0.286
White	62.7%	72.2%	
Black	26.7%	16.7%	
Hispanic	9.3%	5.6%	
All Other	1.3%	5.6%	
Trauma Variables (Possible Score Range)			
Sexual Trauma (0.00-2.00)	0.84 (0.82)	1.47 (0.71)	<0.001
Physical Trauma (0.00-3.00)	0.69 (0.90)	1.56 (1.04)	<0.001
Crime Related Trauma (0.00-4.00)	0.63 (0.73)	3.11 (0.74)	<0.001
General Trauma (0.00-13.00)	3.27 (1.95)	6.75 (2.60)	<0.001
Raped by Sex Partner	12.3%	18.3%	0.319
Raped by Friend/Acquaintance	20.6%	32.4%	0.107
Raped by Stranger	13.7%	35.2%	0.003
Raped by Family Member	18.1%	32.4%	0.048
Psychological Functioning Variables			
Beck Depression Inventory Score	26.2 (12.3)	31.3 (13.5)	0.018
Cutoff for Gen. Anxiety Disorder	66.7%	88.9%	0.001
Cutoff for PTSD	48.0%	90.3%	<0.001
Alcohol Variables			
Any Alcohol Treatment in Prior 90 Days	9.3%	25.0%	0.012
Short Inv. of Problems Score (0-45)	15.70(12.73)	25.26(13.81)	<0.001
Age First Drunk	15.1(4.2)	13.5(4.2)	0.022
Alcohol Consequences Score (0-14)	4.61(3.29)	7.87(3.62)	<0.001
Drug Variables			
Heroin/Opiates in Last 90 Days	5.3%	8.3%	0.470
Cocaine Last 90 Days	52.0%	70.8%	0.019
Age 1st Time Injected (n = 60)	25.1(7.5)	20.5(5.8)	0.012
Drug Injection in Last 90 Days	12.0%	26.4%	0.026
Shared Needle/Works in Last 90 Days	33.3%	84.2%	0.007
Had a Main Partner Who Injected	13.3%	44.4%	<0.001
Crackhouse or Gallery > 1X/Week	17.3%	38.9%	0.004
Any Drug Treatment in Prior 90 Days	12.0%	25.0%	0.042
Ever on Methadone	16.0%	45.8%	<0.001

TABLE 2 (continued)

LCA Variable	Class 1 (n = 75)	Class 2 (n = 72)	p-value
Sex Risk Variables			
Sex for Drugs/Money Last 90 Days	16.0%	31.9%	0.023
No Condom Use in Last 90 Days	30.7%	40.3%	0.223
Lifetime # of Ptns (6 pt scale)	2.8(1.2)	3.5(1.5)	0.004
Medical Variables			
Number Medical Conditions (0-7)	0.8 (0.8)	2.0 (1.5)	<0.001
No Health Insurance	44%	47%	0.695
Dr. or ER Visit in Last 90 Days	60.0%	65.3%	0.509
Social Group Variables			
Tangible Support Score (0-4)	3.0	2.6	0.111
# of HIV + Family Members/Friends	1.3 (3.4)	3.7 (7.3)	0.013
People in Life with Drug/Alcohol Prob. (0-4)	1.6 (1.3)	2.5 (1.4)	<0.001
People in Life Encourage Drinking (0-4)	0.7 (1.0)	1.4 (1.6)	0.002

Note: Means (sd) presented for continuous variables and percentages for categorical variables.

criteria for current PTSD. Women in Class 1 differed significantly with rates of 68% and 48% for GAD and PTSD, respectively.

The Classes were also significantly different from one another on several alcohol and drug related variables. Women in Class 2 were significantly more likely to have been in some form of alcohol treatment in the 90 days prior to incarceration (25%), have a score in the "Medium-High," and to have reported a greater number of alcohol related consequences (mean score of 7.9) compared to Class 1 where 9% had been in alcohol treatment, they were likely to have scored in the "Low" category of the SIP and had a mean score of 4.6 on the alcohol consequences.

In terms of drug use, Class 2 women began injecting drugs at an earlier age (20.5 yrs. vs. 25.1), were significantly more likely to have ever been on methadone (46% vs. 16%), shared either their needle or part of their injection drug equipment in the 90 days prior to incarceration (84% vs. 33%), and to have been to a crack house or shooting gallery one or more times per week in the 90 days prior to incarceration (39% vs. 17%). Additionally, women who were members of Class 2 reported a greater number of lifetime sexual partners and more medical conditions than those in Class 1.

Variables characterizing the Classes' social groups indicated that those in Class 2 have more HIV+ friends and family members (an average of 3.7 vs. 1.3), more people in their lives with drug and or alcohol problems, and more people who encourage their continued drinking than the women with Class 1 memberships.

DISCUSSION

These results revealed two distinct classes with profiles that differ significantly on the number of trauma type exposures, current psychological functioning, alcohol treatment, problems, and consequences, drug histories, sexual risk, medical conditions, and social group characteristics. In all areas, members of Class 2 were significantly more likely to report higher levels of measured variables.

We hypothesized that we would identify classes that were qualitatively distinct in terms of the types of trauma experienced. We originally expected to find the classes discovered would differ by trauma types, with one being more likely to have experienced a particular type, for instance, general trauma, and other or others to have experienced different types, for instance sexual. Contrary to expectation, we found all types of measured trauma in each of our two classes. The question of whether different types of trauma are associated with severe problem behaviors, then, will need to be examined in a wider range of women, including some with lesser trauma exposure.

The latent class analysis did, however, offer support for our hypothesis that the classes would differ *quantitatively* with respect to the number of different trauma type exposures. As an exploratory analysis, we tested one-, two-, and three- class models. It was assumed that a one-class model would not accurately describe the data, however, it was expected there was enough variability for at least a two- class model and possibly a three-class solution based on the likelihood that there could exist classes characterized by: (1) no trauma, (2) some trauma, and (3) extensive trauma. Instead, we found that among a sample of incarcerated women with hazardous drinking levels and HIV risk, there was no class that could be characterized as reporting no trauma exposure. Out of a possible total 22 trauma exposures, the mean of Class 1 was 5.4 and the mean of Class 2 was 12.9. Highlighting the magnitude of trauma among this these women, and finding support for Green et al.'s (2005) study of trauma exposures in this population, only 3 women out of the total 147 reported no trauma exposures.

In addition to probing the extent of trauma type exposures, our analysis revealed several other findings of interest. Compared to previous studies investigating trauma and its effects in the overall population of incarcerated women, we found that women with hazardous drinking levels and current HIV risk had much higher rates of past traumatic experiences, current depression, current generalized anxiety, and post-traumatic symptomatology. For instance, Teplin et al. (1996) found a current PTSD rate of 22.3% in a comparable sample of female, jail detainees. In our study, looking specifically at hazardous drinking and HIV at-risk female jail detainees, Class 1 had a rate of more than twice that, with 48% meeting criteria and in Class 2, all but 10% screened positive for PTSD. Also, contrary to previous findings of very low rates of anxiety disorders among incarcerated women, greater than two-thirds of both our classes met the cutoff criteria for GAD (Teplin et al., 1996). These findings of elevated psychiatric disorders and symptoms that extend into the disorders of extreme stress (DES) features of PTSD within the DSM-IV are evidence that this sub-population of incarcerated women are in tremendous need for effective treatment interventions that address the myriad of problems and mental health needs they are burdened by. The field would benefit by future studies that examine more closely the abuse and trauma dynamics these women experience such as age of onset, frequency of occurrence and relationship to the perpetrator(s). This is especially relevant given that research has indicated that individuals with DES features often have poor PTSD treatment outcomes and that before attempting to treat PTSD, it may be beneficial to address dissociation and interpersonal relationship problems in individuals with DES symptoms (van der Kolk, Roth, Pelcovitz, Sunday, & Spinazzola, 2005).

Our study is not without limitations. Our sample included only female detainees who reported recent hazardous drinking and HIV-risk-taking behaviors. Research has repeatedly shown that past experiences of trauma, especially interpersonal, are related to HIV risk engagement and alcohol and drug use disorders (McNutt et al., 2002; Petrak, Byrne, & Baker, 2000; Whitmire, Harlow, Quina, & Morokoff, 1999), so we were aware that this secondary analysis of a trial enrolling women with these risks would likely reveal high levels of trauma, but we were surprised by the variety and magnitude of past traumatic experiences, as well as the breadth of associated symptoms and risky behaviors. Findings from this sample of the larger female correctional population may not be generalizable to other samples of female detainees who do not have recent HIV and drinking risk behaviors. However, despite the high-risk nature of this population, we believed that it represented a unique opportunity to inform intervention for those potentially most in need and/or most likely to have had trauma exposure.

Additionally, since the study was not designed specifically with identifying trauma classes as a primary outcome, our measures are somewhat limited in terms of allowing us to fully tap the possibility of qualitative differences. We utilized brief "count" measures that are better suited for identifying the quantitative differences and may have contributed to not finding significant qualitative differences of trauma type between the classes. Furthermore, we did not distinguish between childhood and adult trauma exposure and research has found a high correlation between the two with more severe and additional negative outcomes in victims who have experienced trauma throughout the lifespan (Mezey, Bacchus, Bewley, & White, 2005; Whitmire et al., 1999). Also of note, a third of the women in Class 2 reported having been in foster care as a child, evidencing substantial maltreatment within their family of origin. Future directions should incorporate more characteristics of family of origin, as this has been associated with both childhood trauma exposure and later incarceration (Harlow, 1999; Whitmire et al., 1999). It may be that having had more variables assessing added qualitative aspects of trauma might have allowed us to identify classes that differed qualitatively. Due to this current limitation, we cannot justify the exclusion of qualitatively distinct classes.

Finally, we relied on self-report to determine trauma history, sex, alcohol, and drug risk behaviors. It is possible that participants may have been influenced by social desirability and our results may represent underestimates of trauma exposure, sex, alcohol, and drug risk behaviors. However, interviews were conducted in a confidential, unmonitored setting, and research assistants were specially trained to assure participants that their responses would remain confidential.

Despite these limitations, we found support that distinct subgroups of women can be characterized by their number of trauma type exposures within a group of hazardously drinking and HIV at-risk incarcerated women. Future studies can potentially utilize this finding to better tailor interventions and specific program design in hopes of enhancing outcomes with limited service resources. However, given the gravity of measured outcomes across both classes, it is clear that Class 1 participants cannot be dismissed as having no need for trauma services. Instead, future research should examine even more specific differences between the two classes, as different interventions may be useful. For instance, Class 2 reports greater drug risk, with 84.2% of those who inject reporting recent sharing of their drug injection equipment. Studies should also examine if the Classes differ in treatment outcomes based on type of intervention (e.g., cognitive behavioral therapy, therapeutic community) and their trauma exposures.

REFERENCES

Akaike, H. (1981). Likelihood of a model and information criteria. *Journal of Econometrics, 16*, 3-14.

Austin, J., Bloom, B., & Donahue, T. (1992). *Female offenders in the community: An analysis of innovative strategies and programs.* Washington, DC: National Institute of Corrections.

Beck, A. T., Steere, R. A., & Brown, G. K. (1996). *Manual for the Beck Depression Inventory-II.* San Antonio, TX: Psychological Corporation.

Bradley, R. G., & Follingstad, D. R. (2003). Group therapy for incarcerated women who experienced interpersonal violence: a pilot study. *Journal of Traumatic Stress, 16*, 337-340.

Brennan, T., & Austin, J. (1997). *Women in jail: Classification issues.* Washington, DC: National Institute of Corrections.

Browne, A., Miller, B., & Maguin, E. (1999). Prevalence and severity of lifetime physical and sexual victimization among incarcerated women. *International Journal of Law and Psychiatry, 22*, 301-322.

Curtis, R. L., Leung, P., Sullivan, E., Eschbach, K., & Stinson, M. (2001). Outcomes of child sexual contacts: Patterns of incarcerations from a national sample. *Child Abuse & Neglect, 25*, 719-736.

El-Bassel, N., Witte, S. S., Wada, T., Gilbert, L., & Wallace, J. (2001). Correlates of partner violence among female street-based sex workers: substance abuse, history of childhood abuse, and HIV risks. *AIDS Patient Care and STDs, 15*, 41-51.

Epstein, J. N., Saunders, B. E., Kilpatrick, D. G., & Resnick, H. S. (1998). PTSD as a mediator between childhood rape and alcohol use in women. *Child Abuse & Neglect, 22*, 223-234.

Feinn, R., Tennen, H., & Kranzler, H.R. (2003). Psychometric properties of the Short Index of Problems as a measure of recent alcohol-related problems. *Alcoholism: Clinical and Experimental Research, 27*, 1436-1441.

Felitti, V. J., Anda, R. F., Nordenberg, D., Williamson, D. F., Spitz, A. M., Edwards, V., et al. (1998). Relationship of childhood abuse and household dysfunction to many of the leading causes of death in adults. The Adverse Childhood Experiences (ACE) Study. *American Journal of Preventive Medicine, 14*, 245-258.

Gil-Rivas, V., Fiorentine, R., Anglin, M. D., & Taylor, E. (1997). Sexual and physical abuse: Do they compromise drug treatment outcomes? *Journal of Substance Abuse Treatment, 14*, 351-358.

Green, B. (1996). Trauma History Questionnaire. In B. H. Stamm & E. M. Varra (Eds.), *Measurement of stress, trauma, and adaptation* (pp. 366-369). Lutherville, MD: Sidron Press.

Green, B. L., Miranda, J., Daroowalla, A., & Siddique, J. (2005). Trauma exposure, mental health functioning, and program needs of women in jail. *Crime & Delinquency, 51,* 133-151.

Greenfeld, L. A., & Snell, T. L. (1999). *Women offenders* (Bureau of Justice Statistics, NCJ 175688). Washington, DC: U.S. Department of Justice.

Harlow, C. W. (1999). *Prior abuse reported by inmates and probationers* (Bureau of Justice Statistics, NCJ 172879). Washington, DC: U.S. Department of Justice.

Harrison, P. M., & Beck, A. J. (2005). *Prison and jail inmates at midyear 2004* (Bureau of Justice Statistics, NCJ 208801). Washington, DC: U.S. Department of Justice.

Hill, E. M., Blow, F. C., Young, J. P., & Singer, K. M. (1994). Family history of alcoholism and childhood adversity: Joint effects on alcohol consumption and dependence. *Alcoholism: Clinical and Experimental Research, 18,* 1083-1090.

Law Enforcement Assistance Administration. (1998). Women in criminal justice: A twenty year update. Washington, DC: U.S. Department of Justice.

Levin, B. L., Blanch, A. K., & Jennings, A. (1998). *Women's mental health services: A public health perspective.* Thousand Oaks, CA: Sage Publications.

Marquart, J. W., Brewer, V. E., Mullings, J., & Crouch, B. N. (1999). The implications of crime control policy on HIV/AIDS-related risk among women prisoners. *Crime and Delinquency, 45,* 82-96.

McCutcheon, A. L. (1987). *Latent class analysis.* Newbury Park, CA: Sage Publications.

McNutt, L. A., Carlson, B. E., Persaud, M., & Postmus, J. (2002). Cumulative abuse experiences, physical health, and health behaviors. *Annals of Epidemiology, 12,* 123-130.

Messerman-Moore, T. L., & Brown, A. L. (2004). Child maltreatment and perceived family environment as risk factors for adult rape: Is child sexual abuse the most salient experience? *Child Abuse & Neglect, 28,* 1019-1034.

Mezey, G., Bacchus, L., Bewley, S., & White, S. (2005). Domestic violence, lifetime trauma and psychological health of childbearing women. *International Journal of Obstetrics and Gynaecology, 112,* 197-204.

Morash, M., Bynum, T. S., & Koons, B. A. (1998). *Women offenders: Programming needs and promising approaches.* Washington, DC: U.S. Department of Justice, National Institute of Justice.

Mullings, J. L., Marquart, J. W., & Brewer, V. E. (2000). Assessing the relationship between childhood sexual abuse and marginal living conditions on HIV/AIDS-related risk behavior among women prisoners. *Child Abuse & Neglect, 24,* 677-688.

Paone, D., & Chavkin, W. (1993). From the private family domain to the public health forum: Sexual abuse, women, and risk for HIV infection. *SIECUS Report, 21,* 13-15.

Petrak, J., Byrne, A., & Baker, M. (2000). The association between abuse in childhood and STD/HIV risk behaviors in female genitourinary (GU) clinic attendees. *Sexually Transmitted Infections, 76,* 457-461.

Roth, S., Newman, E., Pelcovitz, D., van der Kolk, B., & Mandel, F. (1997). Complex PTSD in victims exposed to sexual and physical abuse: Results from the DSM-IV field trial for posttraumatic stress disorder. *Journal of Traumatic Stress, 10,* 539-555.

Sanders, J. F., & McNeill, K. F. (1997). The incarcerated female felon and substance abuse: Demographics, needs assessment, and program planning for a neglected population. *Journal of Addictions & Offender Counseling, 18,* 41-51.

Schwarz, G. (1978). Estimating the dimension of a model. *Annals of Statistics, 6,* 461-464.

Sherbourne, C. D. & Stewart, A. L. (1991). The MOS Social Support Survey. *Social Science and Medicine, 32,* 705-714.

Teplin, L. A., Abram, K. M., & McClelland, G. M. (1996). Prevalence of psychiatric disorders among incarcerated women: I. Pretrial jail detainees. *Archives of General Psychiatry, 53,* 505-512.

Van der Kolk, B. A., Roth, S., Pelcovitz, D., Sunday, S., & Spinazzola, J. (2005). Disorders of extreme stress: The empirical foundation of a complex adaptation to trauma. *Journal of Traumatic Stress, 18,* 389-399.

Whitmire, L. E., Harlow, L. L., Quina, K., & Morokoff, P. J. (1999). *Childhood trauma and HIV: Women at risk.* New York: Taylor & Francis.

Widom, C. A. (1995). *Victims of childhood sexual abuse–later criminal consequences.* (Bureau of Justice Statistics, NCJ 151525). Washington, DC: U.S. Department of Justice.

Widom, C. A., & Ames, M. A. (1994). Criminal consequences of childhood sexual victimization. *Child Abuse & Neglect, 18,* 303-318.

Zimmerman, M., & Mattia, J. I. (2001a). The Psychiatric Diagnostic Screening Questionnaire: Development, reliability and validity. *Comprehensive Psychiatry, 42,* 175-189.

Zimmerman, M., & Mattia, J. I. (2001b). A self-report scale to help make psychiatric diagnoses. *Archives of General Psychiatry, 58,* 787-794.

Zlotnick, C. (1997). Posttraumatic stress disorder (PTSD), PTSD comorbidity, and childhood abuse among incarcerated women. *Journal of Nervous and Mental Disease, 185,* 761-763.

Zlotnick, C., Najavits, L. M., Rohsenow, D. J., & Johnson, D. M. (2003). A cognitive-behavioral treatment for incarcerated women with substance abuse disorder and posttraumatic stress disorder: Findings from a pilot study. *Journal of Substance Abuse Treatment, 25,* 99-105.

doi:10.1300/J229v08n02_03

Women Domestic Violence Offenders: Lessons of Violence and Survival

Cindy L. Seamans, PhD
Linda J. Rubin, PhD
Sally D. Stabb, PhD

SUMMARY. This qualitative study examined female domestic violence offenders via structured interviews with 13 women referred for treatment in batterers' intervention programs in a major metropolitan area. The majority of women were victims of childhood abuse and/or witnessed violence between their parents. Most reported feeling cut-off from their mothers, left their childhood homes before the age of 18, and experienced violence at the hands of a prior partner. Women's motivations for current violence were primarily in self-defense or in retaliation for their partners' physical abuse, and secondarily in response to partner emotional abuse, control tactics, to get attention/be heard, or to express anger. A minority sought to control their partners. Differential treatment considerations and recommendations

Cindy L. Seamans is affiliated with Texas Woman's University, 6904 Meadow Lake Avenue, Dallas, TX 75214 (E-mail: clseamans@hotmail.com).

Linda J. Rubin, and Sally D. Stabb are affiliated with Texas Woman's University, P.O. Box 425589, Department of Psychology, Denton, TX 76204.

The author gratefully acknowledges Deborah Cosimo and Abhi Kang at The Family Place in Dallas, Texas, and Jennifer Morrison at The New Beginning Center in Garland, Texas for their help and support in working with the participants in this study.

[Haworth co-indexing entry note]: "Women Domestic Violence Offenders: Lessons of Violence and Survival." Seamans, Cindy L., Linda J. Rubin, and Sally D. Stabb. Co-published simultaneously in *Journal of Trauma & Dissociation* (The Haworth Medical Press, an imprint of The Haworth Press, Inc.) Vol. 8, No. 2, 2007, pp. 47-68; and: *Trauma and Dissociation in Convicted Offenders: Gender, Science, and Treatment Issues* (ed: Kathryn Quina, and Laura S. Brown) The Haworth Medical Press, an imprint of The Haworth Press, Inc., 2007, pp. 47-68. Single or multiple copies of this article are available for a fee from The Haworth Document Delivery Service [1-800-HAWORTH, 9:00 a.m. - 5:00 p.m. (EST). E-mail address: docdelivery@haworthpress.com].

Available online at http://jtd.haworthpress.com
doi:10.1300/J229v08n02_04

for women versus men batterers are included. doi:10.1300/J229v08n02_04
[Article copies available for a fee from The Haworth Document Delivery Service: 1-800-HAWORTH. E-mail address: <docdelivery@haworthpress.com> Website: <http://www.HaworthPress.com> © *2007 by The Haworth Press, Inc. All rights reserved.]*

KEYWORDS. Gender, domestic violence, offenders

INTRODUCTION

Increasing numbers of women are being arrested for assaulting their partners, in part due to the trend towards mandatory arrest procedures for partner violence (Hamberger & Potente, 1994; Miller, 2001). Nationwide, women offenders have represented between 5% and 10% of domestic violence related prosecutions (Hooper, 1996). Communities have been advocating the arrest of women either through mandatory dual arrest procedures, in which both parties in a dispute have been arrested (Martin, 1997; Swan & Snow, 2002), or via police policies that have determined victims and perpetrators through surface examinations of which party had visible injuries. While most observers have generally believed that the increase in the number of women arrested for assaulting their partners has been an unintended consequence of mandatory arrest policies created to protect women victims (Swan & Snow, 2002), some have believed it has been a product of an antifeminist backlash (Renzetti, 1997).

Controversy has raged over the conflict between reports of researchers who claimed that wives have assaulted husbands at least as often as husbands have assaulted wives and reports from medical, legal, and social service agencies that women were far more likely to be the victims of domestic assaults (Loeske & Kurz, 2005; Straus, 2005). Moving the discussion about female batterers beyond the who hits whom more often controversy requires a basic understanding of the sources of the data that result in such disparate statistics. Epidemiological studies that have utilized self-report survey data asking intimate partners about conflict in their relationships have reported similar rates of male-to-female and female-to-male inflicted violence (Archer, 2000; Ehrensaft, Moffitt & Caspi, 2005; Fergusson, Horwood & Ridder, 2005; Straus & Gelles, 1986). On the other hand, national crime statistics, crime studies, and hospital emergency room studies have found a much higher percentage of couples in which men were perpetrators and women were victims (Cascardi, Langhinrichsen, & Vivian, 1992; Goodyear-Smith & Laidlaw, 1999; Rennison, 2003; Straus, 1999).

While the proportion of male to female perpetrators was much higher in crime studies than family conflict studies, the incident rate of violent episodes perpetrated by either gender was much lower in crime studies and in police statistics than in family conflict studies. In a review, Straus (1999) noted that family conflict studies reported an annual assault rate ranging from 10% to 35% and averaging 16%. By contrast, the National Violence Against Women study (Tjaden & Thoennes, 1997) reported a 1.1% annual assault rate.

Some researchers and theorists (Johnson, 1995, 2005; Swan & Snow, 2002) have suggested that the couple-conflict studies and battered women advocates were coming in contact with two completely different phenomena. Johnson (1995) stated that couple-conflict studies described "common couple violence," a more gender-neutral phenomenon in which "conflict occasionally gets out of hand leading usually to minor forms of violence and more rarely escalating into serious, sometimes even life-threatening forms of violence" (p. 2). On the contrary, battered women advocates were coming in contact with a much less common phenomenon, that of patriarchal terrorism by husbands over wives, "the systematic use of not only violence, but economic subordination, threats, isolation and other control tactics" (Johnson, 1995, p. 2).

Many researchers and theorists have claimed that most women who used violent behavior with their partners did so in self-defense or as a peremptory strike to prevent being harmed (Dasgupta, 1999; Hamberger & Guse, 2002; Hamberger, Lohr, & Bonge,1994; Henning, Jones, & Holdford, 2005; Miller & Meloy, 2005; Watson, 2000). Some of the reasons for violence that emerged from the interviews with the women in these studies were retaliation for past violence or emotional abuse, self-defense, and escape from being restrained or from a situation perceived as threatening. Additionally, some women became violent as an expressive act after becoming frustrated by being abandoned or ignored.

While the men have not endorsed self-defense or retaliation for past physical abuse, they have talked about punishing their partners' past bad behaviors and the need to physically control their partners (Hamberger et al., 1994). Countless male and female domestic violence offenders have described a pattern of conflict arising, men trying to leave, women trying to continue the dialogue by preventing the men from leaving, and violence erupting. Both genders also have endorsed anger expression as an important reason for their violent behaviors (Hamberger et al., 1994;

Jack, 1999). For men, the need to stop their partners' expressions of anger (e.g., "shut her up") also has emerged as a reason to become violent (Hamberger et al., 1994).

Both Campbell (1993) and Jack (1999) described women's aggression in terms of a loss of control. Jack points out that many women do not feel in charge of themselves when engaging in aggressive acts. "Instead they feel passive, as if 'it' made me do it ... As these women fail to 'control' their aggression, they observe themselves both as subject to the feeling of rage and as the one who was unable to control it" (p. 177). Those who may have PTSD may be prone to such dissociative states (van der Hart, Nijenhuis, & Steele, 2005).

Experiencing childhood trauma including childhood sexual and physical abuse has been linked to post traumatic stress disorder (PTSD) and to dissociation (Collin-Vezina & Hebert, 2005; Stovall-McClough & Cloitre, 2006). In a recent study of female survivors, Kubiak (2006) found that unresolved childhood sexual abuse was associated with a 7.5 fold increase in the likelihood of being diagnosed with PTSD. The cumulative effects of multiple childhood traumas have been shown to exponentially affect the likelihood of suffering from dissociation and PTSD as an adult. Kubiak (2005) found that the odds of suffering from PTSD increased 40% with each added traumatic event or category.

By and large, women batterers have been court-referred into domestic violence treatment programs that were established to intervene with male perpetrators. How has this fit for them? Were women who physically attacked their male partners motivated by the same paradigm of power and control (Pence & Paymar, 1993) that many theorists and researchers have claimed has motivated male batterers? Or were they striking out in response to or in anticipation of male violence? Have women used violence against their partners as a way of expressing their feelings rather than as a tactic of power and control? Have women batterers had the same characteristics and history of abuse as male batterers? This study was designed to shed light on some of these questions.

METHODOLOGY

Participants

This study was conducted with 13 women perpetrators of domestic violence who had sought counseling at urban battering intervention programs. The number of participants was determined based on data analyses, with interviews continuing until saturation (Glaser & Strauss, 1967) that is, until no substantially new data or themes emerged. These women were either court-referred into counseling following an arrest for domestic violence on charges that included assault and aggravated assault with a deadly weapon or were referred to the programs by the Texas Department of Child Protective Services (CPS).

Most of the participants were quite young, with a mean age of 28. All women were married or cohabiting with their partners. The majority of the women in this study (54%) reported moving out of their family of origin homes before the age of 18, subsequently moving in with abusive men. Four of the women had partners of a different race. The 21% inter-racial marriage rate of these participants was four times higher than the national average (Fletcher, 1998). Four of the women were not employed outside of their homes at the time of their referrals into the programs. The remaining eight had diverse types of employment, with four general office workers, an exotic dancer, a tattoo artist, a paralegal, and a telephone operator. Seven of the women were living with children of their own, one was living with a step child, and the remaining four had no children.

Procedure

The participants were recruited by offering women in the perpetrator treatment programs the opportunity to anonymously participate in a structured interview that was tape-recorded and subsequently transcribed and content analyzed for themes. There was no requirement that the women participate in order to receive the counseling services at either of the agencies. The participants were informed in writing of the purpose of the study and given an information packet, including a consent form that outlined the purpose of the study and the procedures taken to ensure the anonymity of the responses. For their participation, each of the women received a $10 gift certificate to Target.

An interview guide was prepared with questions that were open-ended and flexible, designed to elicit detailed information about the women's feelings, attitudes, and behaviors. The research project was conducted from the feminist perspective (Griffin, 1991), with the goal to empower and give voice to the respondents (Gilligan, 1982; Jack, 1999). As a part of this interactive process and as a key form of triangulation, member checks from these participants were obtained.

RESULTS AND DISCUSSION

The richness and depth of the interviews led to findings far beyond the scope of the preliminary research questions. The violence these women perpetrated did not spring from the blue–for most of them it was just another chapter in a lifetime of experience with violence and abuse. Nine major themes from the interview content analysis are presented here. For each, examples are given and links to the literature on both men and women offenders are noted. As is typical for qualitative research, results and discussion are considered together.

Theme One: Childhood Abuse

All women experienced some form of abuse during childhood. Types of abuse are detailed in Table 1.

Of the women who had been physically abused, six out of the seven reported that their mothers or stepmother had been physically abusive to them, while five reported childhood physical abuse by their fathers or stepfathers. Beyond the numbers, the women's stories of physical abuse at the hands of their parents varied in severity, from occasionally being struck with a belt as "discipline," to being traumatized and terrified. Four of the same women also reported being sexually abused as children, two by uncles, one by a stepfather, and one by a stepfather as well as biological father. Becky talked of being impacted as much by her adopted mother's disbelief as she was by her adopted father's abuse.

> I was sexually, mentally, and emotionally abused ... My dad started to abuse me when I was about eight years old ... After I told her (mother) what my dad did to me, she didn't believe me. In fact, she slapped me.

TABLE 1. Childhood abuse history

Type of Abuse	Percent of Participants Endorsing Abuse
Physical abuse by father	38%
Physical abuse by mother	54%
Sexual abuse	31%
Psychological abuse/neglect	85%
Observing parental violence	54%
Disconnected from mother	77%

Almost all women reported childhood psychological abuse or neglect, with six of the women growing up in chaotic households with parents who committed crimes, abused drugs and alcohol, and exposed their daughters to their sexual promiscuity. Jenny told about experiencing and seeing more than any child should witness. "My mother was very, very promiscuous. I walked in on sex acts happening ... I saw her really messed up on drugs, valium and drunk. She passed me a joint when I was nine."

In other cases, the abuse took the form of neglect, with parents who were depressed, self-absorbed, or overwhelmed with the conflict in their own relationships. Ten of the 13 women reported feeling disconnected or cut-off from their mothers, while four said they were estranged from their fathers. Feeling abandoned by parents was a theme woven throughout a number of the interviews.

Susan, who described a middle-class childhood, talked of being abandoned by her parents, rejected after the birth of her siblings. "When I was 13, I got a new brother and sister. We're 10 and 13 years apart. When my brother and sister came along, when I was 13, my mom and dad decided they had their hands full. And kind of, gave me up to the courts."

Watson (2000) was one of the only researchers of female domestic violence offenders who addressed childhood maltreatment, and found that 100% of her participants experienced childhood physical abuse, while 70% of them witnessed interparental violence. With the exception of sexual abuse, these experiences with childhood abuse mirrored the formative years of male batterers (Bevan & Higgins, 2002).

Five of the women reported that their mothers were violent with their fathers or stepfathers, all but one in self-defense, or in response to fathers' violence. Six of the women reported their fathers or stepfathers were violent towards their mothers. Misty talked about finally leaving her mother's home after several chaotic years watching her mother being abused.

> And I remember seeing a boyfriend of hers actually holding her up against the wall by her neck, exactly like David did to me one time ... I thought he was going to kill her. I remember that, being five years old.

For Belinda, it seemed important for her to remember her mother's culpability in her parents' violent exchanges.

> It wasn't the typical husband comes home drunk and beats on his wife. It was more like they would get into a screaming match and

someone would swing. From my memories, it was a very mutual type of thing … I remember standing in between them and screaming for them to stop.

How did witnessing parental violence influence these women in their intimate relationships? For some of these women witnessing parental violence may have normalized spousal violence, making it easier for them to tolerate abuse, or to become abusive themselves. Keisha, whose mother was abused and did not fight back, believed her parents' violence had a major impact on her behavior. "Since I saw her being beat up, I thought it was OK, it was part of the relationship."

For others, seeing their mothers' examples, as victims and as perpetrators, may have been the impetus for choosing to use violence with intimate partners. A recurring pattern in these women's stories was a resolve to refuse to be victims. In some instances, these women's mothers verbally instructed their daughters not to tolerate abuse; in other cases, the women came to the conclusion themselves, based on their own observations of their mothers' suffering.

Misty reported that at age 16 she chose a man much like her abusive stepfather, relying on her childhood experiences in responding to his abuse. "My mom always taught me, don't ever let no man push around on you. And that's when I started standing up for myself, basically.… I always told myself, I'll never have a man hit me …"

Perhaps related to their childhood experiences with violence, and their feelings about their parents, seven of the women reported leaving their childhood homes before age 18. Eleven out of 13 of these women reported varying degrees of disconnect in their relationships with their mothers. All of the women whose mothers were physically abusive to them stated feeling estranged from their mothers, including those who reported childhood sexual abuse. Ten of the 11 who talked of feeling disconnected or estranged from their mothers also reported childhood psychological abuse or neglect. All of the women whose mothers were the victims of their fathers' or stepfathers' violence felt estranged from their mothers.

Leaving home at a young age may be related to women's subsequent experiences with violence, putting them at risk for being preyed upon by abusive men. While five made other choices initially, six out of seven who left home at a young age ended up living with abusive men before their 18th birthdays. The 7th moved in with an extremely abusive man at age 19. Hungry for love and connection, the five who moved out to other homes gravitated quickly to partners who became violent. Other studies have linked early cohabitation to domestic violence (Moffitt & Caspi, 1999) and intimate homicide (Rodriguez & Henderson, 1993).

Mothers seemed to take the brunt of their daughters' blame for childhood abuse and violence. While the women described their fathers' abuse, drug use, or abandonment, it was their mothers for whom they reserved the greatest scorn.

Many of these women spent years watching their mothers absorb this pain, with their mothers sometimes becoming depressed, sometimes turning to alcohol or drugs, sometimes fighting back or becoming violent themselves. It was not surprising that these women distanced themselves from their mothers, taking an oath to not be anything like their mothers, and most of all, not to be a victim. And for these women, not being a victim often translated into becoming violent with their partners when they felt threatened.

Jack (1999) summarized the psychological experience of women who felt they were abandoned as children and then became violent to their intimate partners when they threatened to leave as externalizing the "... psychological experience of being destroyed" (p. 162). The same phenomenon may have existed in males who experienced childhood abandonment and neglect, and became violent with their partners when they feared fresh abandonment. Jacobson and Gottman (1998) attributed the motivation of "pit bulls" (p. 64), the group that includes 80% of all batterers, to an inability to sustain attachment and a fear of being abandoned by their partners.

But for men, power and violence were congruent with their approved role in society, while for women, becoming violent came at a greater cost, as they acted out of role, incongruent with societal proscriptions. As Gilbert (2002) wrote in her discussion of female violence and gender stereotypes, women who were violent were generally labeled as mad or bad in this society. Our sense of these women was that, for the most part, they were neither mad nor bad. They were desperate.

Theme Two: Prior Partner Violence

Most of the women in this study reported that their prior partners physically abused them. Very few studies of female domestic violence offenders have examined the violence in their previous relationships, instead focusing narrowly on the violent interchanges within their current relationships. Miller (2001) and Dasgupta (1999) reported most of their female domestic violence offenders had been involved with multiple abusive partners.

Regarding prior relationship violence, the majority of the women in the sample (7; 54%) reported physical violence in their past intimate relationships. Only two of the seven reported that they returned their prior partners' violence with aggression of their own.

It was clear that the context that sets the stage for these women who were violent to their partners extended far beyond the dynamics of their current relationships to include their previous relationships as well as their childhoods. For example, Keisha, whose current husband had never been violent to her in any way, was the victim of very serious physical abuse by multiple previous partners, not to mention physical and sexual abuse by her parents. She came into her current relationship a trauma victim, perhaps suffering from PTSD, and became violent with her current husband while in the throes of post-partum depression. Several authors reported that women perpetrators of domestic violence exhibit symptoms of PTSD (Abel, 1999; O'Keefe, 1998). The origin of these women's PTSD symptoms may lie not in their current relationships, but in prior adult abusive relationships or in childhood abuse.

Damaged goods or merely resilient and resourceful, they learned from their past violent relationships that sitting back and taking it did not stop the violence. These women entered their current relationships near the ends of their ropes, with little tolerance for enduring abuse.

Theme Three: Current Partner Violence

The women in the study endorsed a number of reasons for resorting to violence with their current partners, with eight (62%) claiming they were responding in self-defense or in an attempt to retaliate.

Kate, a former high school athlete, told of enduring her partner's escalating violence for many months before finally responding with violence.

> For the longest time, he would more or less hit me. And I just let him do it ... I just finally got fed up with it, and I'd bite him, or I'd try to kick him, just to get away ... How would I get a charge for assault when everything I did was out of self defense?

Tonya had experienced severe abuse from a prior partner, as well as past abuse from her husband before the exchange that resulted in her arrest when she grabbed a weapon to help even the playing field.

> ... When all this happened, he had a warrant out for his arrest for ... physically hitting me and stuff like that ... We started arguing, and then he hit me, and then I hit him back.... I got the knife. I was

just trying to scare him. I just did like this, (holds hand out) and I didn't know I stabbed him.... I guess I was just defending myself.

Several of the women spoke of fighting back not solely because they feared their partner or his abuse, but because they refused to see themselves as victims. Belinda described responding to her husband's violence for years until her marriage evolved into a tumultuous setting of mutual combat. A large, strong woman, Belinda appeared proud that she could give as well as she could get. "And he always knew, that I knew, that he could kill me. But he knew that I would go down fighting."

In addition to fighting back in self-defense, some of the women reported being violent to their partners in retaliation for a range of abusive behaviors, including physical abuse, being restrained or confined, verbal abuse, and psychological abuse. Five of the women said their partners tried to physically keep them from leaving, and, in some instances, they responded to that restraint by lashing out with physical violence. Jenny described a typical interchange.

He was laying on top of me, holding me down, because ... I wanted to run away ... and I was screaming at him, "get off me now, get off me." And he wouldn't get off me. And I reached up and I bit him in his nose, And he reached down and he bit me back.

Other studies of women domestic violence perpetrators confirmed that self-defense was an important motivating factor for the majority of women who were violent to their partners (Dasgupta, 1999; Hamberger & Guse, 2002; Swan & Snow, 2002; Watson, 2000). Men also were likely to become perpetrators of partner violence when they had been a victim of abuse, particularly when they had experienced severe physical abuse at the hands of their partners (Makepeace, 1986).

With the typical strength differential between the sexes, women may be less able to inflict injury on their male partners with a casual slap or shove, but can be dangerous when they hurl objects or use weapons. Most of the women in this study (8 out of 13) stated they have thrown things at their partners and five of them admitted to using weapons against their intimate partners. When women used these behaviors, violence often escalated, as their partners responded with equal or greater force.

When women used violence, they were acting outside the bounds of their typical gender role (Campbell, 1993). These women looked nothing like helpless victims when the police arrived. These women had internalized a commitment to not being victims, and they were more likely to be labeled by police officers as crazy or dangerous, resulting in their arrests.

Theme Four: Retaliation for Emotional Abuse

The majority (8; 62%) reported that psychological that sometimes incited them to retaliate with physical violence. The most extreme example of that response was Marge, whose husband had been constantly emotionally, but not physically, abusive to her during their 19-year marriage.

> Oh, he would call me stupid, gordo, which means fatso. He called me, what really hurt so bad was when he called me his $10 slave ... I had asked him, why did he call me that? And he said, "Well, that's what I paid for you when I married you." Oh, my God. I was doing his laundry, and I yelled down the hall, "Will you come down here and put up your good clothes so they won't get wrinkled?" And he said, "No, that's what I got my $10 slave for." That just got me more madder ... So, I hung up his clothes, and I just happened to look up on the shelf.... and I saw his (gun) ... And I picked it up ... I didn't know that the thing was cocked, or anything ... Before I could even get any words out, it went off. Scared me to death.

Marge was arrested that night for shooting her husband in the head while he was lying down on the couch with his back turned to her. While Marge was not surprised to be arrested, Nancy was shocked when she was arrested for slapping her husband in retaliation for his emotional abuse.

> He said, how did he put it? "I've been thinking about my ex-wife and all of her redeeming qualities ... none of which you could aspire to." I turned around and slapped him.... And maybe part of it was just turning around and going, no, it's inappropriate. I'm not powerless.

Maria's partner was physically, as well as emotionally, abusive to her, but it was the verbal abuse that inspired her to strike him.

> I mean when a man calls you a cunt and a whore in front of your kids, no matter how young they were, it does something to you ... It would just enrage me until I would tell him, "You can't be doing that or I'm going to knock the shit out of you."

Theme Five: Violence and Children

One of the most unexpected findings of this study was the apparent connection between being mothers of infants and being domestic violence offenders. Thirty-eight percent (five) of the women mention their violence in the context of the birth of their children. For these women, having a new baby may have pushed them to a breaking point, the end of the rope that most of the women mention when describing why they chose to lash out physically against their current partners. Two of the women specifically said they believed they were suffering from untreated post-partum depression when they committed the violent acts that led to their arrests. Both of these women had recently given birth to twins.

> Keisha described her feelings, "I was scared of coming home and taking care of the babies by myself.... I thought I was not going to be a good mother. I thought I couldn't take care of two by myself. I just cried."

Cut off from their mothers, and tired from the 24-hour demands of their infants, these women reached the breaking point. Behaviors they may have tolerated earlier, such as drug use or verbal abuse, were no longer acceptable.

Theme Six: Asking for Help and Not Getting It and the Mandatory Arrest Policy

If most of these women were victims of abuse, who were fighting back or retaliating for physical and emotional maltreatment, why did they not ask for help, and flee these relationships, rather than becoming violent? Perhaps part of the answer lies in their youth, and the fact that many of them fled abusive childhood homes, only to find abusive partners. Other women described trying to call the police, but being physically restrained by their partners, or having their partners tear the telephones out of the wall to prevent them calling the police. But many of these women did ask for help, from their families, from their partners' families, and from the police, only to be rebuffed and arrested.

Seven of the women reported unsuccessfully reaching out for help, either in this relationship, or in prior violent relationships, more often than not, calling the police because they were afraid for their safety resulted in being arrested themselves. Additionally, several of the women said calling the police was not an option because of their partners' connections to law enforcement, or the power of their monetary influence. Men also were becoming increasingly savvy about manipulating the criminal justice system to control their partners.

The lack of a support system, and the inability to turn to family members for help, may be one of the most critical threads that ran throughout the fabric of these women's violent and abusive lives. Several mention turning to family members when violence erupted in their households, only to be rejected.

Theme Seven: Power and Control

If battering was a coercive pattern of power and control, then it was important to examine how control issues played a role in the conflicts and violence in these women's relationships. Rather than who hit whom, how many times, and who was now bleeding, the questions from this perspective were: Who was afraid, and who was in control?

Only two (15%) of the women in this study reported trying to control their partners as part of their motivation for becoming violent. Both of these women described their relationships as mutual struggles for control, with their partners also attempting to exert control over them. Both women described their partners as larger and stronger, and said they were often afraid of them.

Some of the women in Dasgupta's (1999) study also said that they used violence to gain control of situations. Watson (2000) specifically asked her participants, "Do female perpetrators use physical violence to gain dominance, power, and control or were there different purposes?" (p. 55). Only one of the 10 participants acknowledged that her own motivation was primarily to control her partner.

Additionally, many women in these studies said that their partners tried to exert control over them, and that resisting their partners' control led to violence in their homes. Eight of 13 (62%) women in this study reported that their partners were controlling, using various tactics to exert power over them including: limiting or stealing money; physically blocking the door, blocking in her car, taking her keys, and/or disabling her car; isolating her from family, friends, or activities; refusing to let her use the phone and/or pulling the phone out of the wall; monitoring her behavior, checking up on her, searching her purse; demanding dinner at a specific time; confiscating passports, threatening pets, threatening children and other family members and/or threatening to call the police.

The men in these women's lives used fear and intimidation to try to control them. Eight of the 13 women reported fearing their partners. Even Belinda, who found it so important to be brave and to stand up and give as much as she got, admitted she feared her partner. "I always knew if he could kill me if he hit me the wrong way or the right way whichever way you want to look at it. . . . And he loves that power. He thrives on power."

Most of the women (7, 54%) said their partners' jealousy was the underlying cause of their controlling behavior, which lead to the violence in their relationships. None of the women mentioned being jealous of their partners. An eighth woman described the events leading up to shooting her husband as starting with his anger at being denied sexual access. Misty said her partner broke her arm during an argument over her supposed infidelity. Jenny said her partner was jealous, not only of other men, but also of any attention she gave to anyone else.

Evolutionary psychologists believe domestic violence emerged from the need of males to control female sexuality in order to assure their paternity. Therefore, as Peters, Shackelford, and Buss (2002) found in their recent analysis, domestic violence was almost universally perpetrated on young women of childbearing age. The age range of the women in the study, 19-42 years old, places all of them in their childbearing years.

Theme Eight: Violence Motivated by the Need to Be Heard

While control was rarely a goal, many of these women were driven by the need to get their partner's attention. Nine (69%) of the women said they were frustrated and enraged by their partner's refusal to talk about problems. These women said they were moved to violence when their partners ignored them, or left.

Belinda described desperately needing her partner to listen to her, and fearing that if her partner was allowed to leave an argument, he would abandon her and their relationship. This desperation was reminiscent of her descriptions of her childhood, when her father abandoned the family, and she and her mother would drive the streets searching for him.

> I mean, his answer for everything was walking away from it. Mine was full-on, head-on confrontation. Damn it, you're going to listen to me if I have to tie your ass down, and, you know, gag you, you're going to listen to me.

Nancy described feeling desperate to communicate with both past and current partners. She believes this cycle of pursuing men when they want to shut down was typical of all women's behaviors. "I want to talk about it so badly ... I think that's what females have, a tendency to do that. Males feel cornered, attacked.

Campbell (1993) believes that men's and women's aggression is different, that men use aggression instrumentally to gain control over another person or to gain social and material benefits, while women use aggression expressively, as a "cry for help born out of desperation" (p. 7). Campbell's ideas are supported by the interview data in this study.

Looking at the bigger picture, perhaps these women were particularly prone to becoming affronted by their partners disregard because of their own childhood abuse and neglect. The messages of unworthiness these women internalized as children may have set them up for being particularly reactive to partners who neglect or ignore them. For the women in this study, when their partners shut down and ignore them, it pours gasoline on the fires of their insecurities, setting up spirals of escalating rage and violence.

Theme Nine: Reaching the Breaking Point

The majority of these women, seven (54%) described becoming enraged and losing control of themselves. While they often described their partners' violence as tools they use to control them, the women described their own violence as a loss of control, a response almost out of their cognitive awareness.

Belinda has struck her mother, and girlfriends, as well as her husband. She described the feelings of rage that engulfed her. "I mean, honestly, if I was, God forbid, if I ever seriously hurt somebody, my lawyer could actually go for temporary insanity because during that time, during the act of violence, I am not there. I am somewhere else."

Heather was incredulous at the damage she had inflicted on her stepson. " I thought I only hit him five times, and then the pictures came out. And it was like, no, ... you hit him so many times, it's hard to count. Were you in a rage? Did you black out?... I must have been in such a rage that I don't remember."

Theme Ten: Posttraumatic Stress Disorder and Dissociative States

In addition to apparently dissociating when they became violent, several of the women reported blocking out other memories, perhaps due to

Posttraumatic Stress Disorder. Belinda reported memory lapses for times she was victimized during her childhood as well as with her violent partner. "I have this gift of blocking things out that are traumatic, so it is hard to remember a lot of the details. These are only tiny memories and I know there's been more. And I only remember that because my mom brought it up to me."

Many of the women in this study experienced multiple childhood traumas that could have created traumatic stress reactions. For many, childhood physical and/or sexual abuse was later followed by growing up to participate as a victim, perpetrator, or both in partner violence. Grella, Stein and Greenwell's (2005) recent study of childhood trauma in substance-abusing women offenders linked early experiences with traumatic events such as serious accidents and death of a close family member to engaging in violent crime. Several of the women in the present study were poster children for childhood trauma, including Susan, whose traumatic experiences began when she was four, and included surviving a car accident that killed her brother and another child, and then subsequent placement in foster care. She called her dissociative states when fighting with her current partner "blackouts." "I've beaten him unmercifully and not even known I'd done it … I don't know what happened. I snapped."

Jenny lost a limb to a traumatic injury as a child, and also experienced her childhood home burning down to be followed by witnessing horrendous inter-parental violence. She said her childhood made her very wary, and perhaps hypervigilant, to perceived threats.

Becky reported blaming the overwhelming feelings of fear she experienced when she tried to have normal sexual interactions with her partner directly on her childhood sexual abuse. "He (her partner) hates my dad with a passion because he just can't be intimate with me. . . . Sometimes I'll think about it (the childhood abuse) and I'll push him away."

IMPLICATIONS FOR INTERVENTION AND TREATMENT

Regardless of history or motivation, most women batterers will be placed on probation and remanded for treatment in batterer intervention programs originally designed for male perpetrators. While there is emerging criticism (Stuart, 2005) of these programs designed around the paradigm of male perpetrator power and control over female victims (Pence & Paymar, 1993), they remain the norm for most court-mandated treatment. It is at the treatment level that society as a whole, and women perpetrators and victims of domestic violence individually, can be better served with more appropriate interventions.

This study explored the specific and nuanced ways that men and women domestic violence offenders were alike and different in their history of childhood abuse, prior partner relationships and motivation for current violence. Nine themes were identified from the interviews with these women offenders including childhood abuse, prior partner violence, current partner violence, retaliation for emotional abuse, violence and children, asking for help and not getting it, power and control, violence motivated by the need to be heard and reaching the breaking point. While there were many similarities between the experiences of women and men batterers, gender differences clearly were demonstrated. Recommendations for treating domestic violence offenders are noted below and emerge from the clear ways in which men's and women's violence are different.

1. *Refer women arrested for domestic violence to groups specifically designed and created for women domestic violence offenders.* Placing women in programs designed to confront patriarchal attitudes and male privilege is ludicrous, yet it is done every day. An even greater disservice is given to women and men who are placed in mixed-gender groups.

2. *Screen women who enter domestic violence treatment programs thoroughly for substance abuse and psychiatric disorders.* A significant number of both male and female perpetrators of domestic violence have substance abuse problems (Kantor & Jasinski, 1998) and should be referred for substance abuse treatment, either in advance of, or concurrent with, the intervention for domestic violence. Women entering domestic violence treatment programs should also be screened carefully for psychiatric disorders, especially Depression, Post-Partum Depression, Post-Traumatic Stress Disorder, and other Anxiety Disorders, with appropriate referrals given for medication evaluations and/or counseling.

3. *Assess the safety level of the woman entering programs, and continue to monitor their living situations for safety and security.* Most women who enter batterers' treatment programs are victims of domestic violence who have survived by believing that they are not victims, that by standing up for themselves, even with violence, they can protect themselves from abuse. Even in the face of long histories of being injured by their partners, many women in batterers' programs are in denial about the level of their own risk. In addition to one-on-one screening, safety planning is an appropriate topic to address in a group

setting, to provide a reality check to members through the feedback of their peers.

4. *Provide appropriate referrals to victim services.* Some social service agencies have the policy of denying victim services to clients who are enrolled in batterers' treatment programs. Women who are perpetrators, but also victims of domestic violence, should be given access to services for victims, including shelter services.

5. *Provide services to children of women referred to batterer treatment programs.* The children of women enrolled in batterers' programs most often have been the victims of domestic violence themselves, either vicariously, through seeing their mothers or fathers abused, or directly, as victims of abuse and neglect. Intervening with their children is an important step to halting the intergenerational transmission of violence.

6. *Provide stress management and anxiety reduction training.* Cognitive-behavioral interventions that focus on combinations of exposure, relaxation techniques, controlled breathing, and positive imagery have been found to be effective in helping individuals with traumatic stress symptoms. Targeting maladaptive beliefs related to safety, trust, and self-esteem are likewise recommended (Hollon & Beck, 2004).

7. *Provide training in anger management techniques.* Assisting women in recognizing the triggers for their anger may be helpful. Once awareness of these cues is established, women can learn a variety of alternative, effective, and non-violent means for expressing their anger. Anger can be recognized as a vital and important emotion while options for adaptive expression are encouraged (Cox, Stabb, & Bruckner, 1999).

8. *Treat the effects of abuse with a strength-based model.* Most women in batterers' treatment programs have been victims of multiple kinds of abuse, yet also have a resilience and resourcefulness that can be tapped for treatment. In fighting back, these women had chosen a dysfunctional way to empower themselves, but treatment providers can redirect this resilience onto more productive paths.

CONCLUSION

It is hoped that the stories of these women and this analysis can shed light on this murky topic. These women, and their sisters still living in pain and violence, deserve more than the reductionist solutions served up by the criminal justice system to their complex problems. Only by embracing their complexity and the contradictions of being both victims and perpetrators can advocates and service providers lead these brave and resilient women out of violence.

REFERENCES

Abel, E. M. (1999). Comparing women in batterer intervention programs with male batterers and female domestic violence victims. (Doctoral dissertation, Case Western Reserve University, 1999). *Dissertation Abstracts International, 60, 07A, 2675.*

Archer, J. (2000). Sex differences in aggression between heterosexual partners: A meta-analytic review. *Psychological Bulletin, 126,* 651-680.

Bevan, E., & Higgins, D. (2002). Is domestic violence learned? The contribution of five forms of child maltreatment to men's violence and adjustment. *Journal of Family Violence, 17,* 223-245.

Campbell, A. (1993). *Men, women and aggression.* New York: BasicBooks.

Cascardi, M., Langhinrichsen, J., & Vivian, D. (1992). Marital aggression: impact, injury, and health correlates for husbands and wives. *Archives of Internal Medicine, 152,* 1178-1184.

Collin-Vezina, D., & Hebert, M. (2005). Comparing dissociation and PTSD in sexually abused school-aged girls. *The Journal of Nervous and Mental Disease, 193,* 47-52.

Cox, D., Stabb, S. D., & Bruckner, K. (1999). *Women's anger: Clinical and developmental perspectives.* Philadelphia: Brunner/Mazel:Taylor & Francis Group.

Dasgupta, S. D. (1999). Just like men? A critical view of violence by women. In M. Shepard & E. Pence, (Eds.), *Coordinating community responses to domestic violence: Lessons from Duluth and beyond* (pp. 195-222). Thousand Oaks, CA: Sage.

Ehrensaft, M., Moffitt, T., & Caspi, A. (2004). Clinically abusive relationships in an unselected birth cohort. Men's and women's participation and developmental antecedents. *Journal of Abnormal Psychology, 113, 2,* 258-270.

Fergusson, D., Horwood, L. J., & Ridder, E. (2005). Partner violence and mental health outcomes in a New Zealand birth cohort. *Journal of Marriage and Family, 67,* 1103-1117.

Fletcher, M. (1998, December 28). Interracial marriages eroding barriers. *The Washington Post,* p. A1.

Gilbert, P. (2002). Discourses of female violence and societal gender stereotypes. *Violence Against Women, 8,* 1271-1300.

Gilligan, C. (1982). *In a different voice. 2nd ed.* Cambridge, MA: Harvard University Press.

Glaser, B., & Strauss, A. (1967). *The discovery of grounded theory: Strategies for qualitative research.* Chicago: Aldine.

Goodyear-Smith, F. A., & Laidlaw, T. M. (1999). Aggressive acts and assaults in intimate relationships: Towards an understanding of the literature. *Behavioral Sciences and the Law, 17,* 285-304.

Grella, C., Stein, J., & Greenwell, L. (2005). Associations among childhood trauma, adolescent problem behaviors, and adverse adult outcomes in substance-abusing women offenders. *Psychology of Addictive Behaviors, 19,* 43-53.

Griffin, C. (1991). The researcher talks back. Dealing with power relations in studies of young people's entry into the job market. In W. Shaffir & R. Stebbins (Eds.) *Experiencing fieldwork* (pp. 109-119). London: Sage Publications.

Hamberger, L. K., & Guse, C. (2002). Men's and women's use of intimate partner violence in clinical samples. *Violence Against Women, 8,* 1301-1331.

Hamberger, L. K., Lohr, J. M., & Bonge, D. (1994). The intended function of domestic violence is different for male and female perpetrators. *Family Violence and Sexual Assault Bulletin, 10,* 40-44.

Hamberger, L. K., & Potente, T. (1994). Counseling heterosexual women arrested for domestic violence: Applications for theory and practice. *Violence and Victims, 9,* 89-137.

Henning, K., Jones, A., & Holdford, R. (2005). "I didn't do it, but if I did I had a good reason": Minimization, denial and attributions of blame among male and female domestic violence offenders. *Journal of Family Violence, 20,* 131-139.

Hollon, S. D., & Beck, A. T. (2004). Cognitive and cognitive-behavioral therapies. In M. J. Lambert (Ed.). *Bergin and Garfield's handbook of psychotherapy and behavior change*, pp. 447-492, New York, NY: Wiley.

Hooper, M. (1996). When domestic violence diversion is no longer an option: What to do with the female offender. *Berkeley Women's Law Journal, 6,* 168-181.

Jack, D. (1999). *Behind the mask. Destruction and creativity in women's aggression.* Cambridge, MA: Harvard University Press.

Jacobson, N., & Gottman, J. (1998). Violent relationship. *Psychology Today,* March/April, 61-84.

Johnson, M. P. (1995). Patriarchal terrorism and common couple violence: Two forms of violence against women. *Journal of Marriage & the Family, 57,* 283-294.

Johnson, M. P. (2005). Domestic violence: It's not about gender–or is it? *Journal of Marriage and Family, 67,* 1126-1130.

Kantor, G. K., & Jasinski, J. L. (1998). Dynamics and risk factors in partner violence. In J. L. Jasinski & L. M. Williams (Eds.) *Partner violence. A comprehensive review of 20 years of research* (pp. 1-72). Thousand Oaks, CA: Sage Publications.

Kubiak, S. (2005). Trauma and cumulative adversity in women of a disadvantaged social location. *American Journal of Orthopsychiatry, 75,* 451-465.

Loseke, D. R., & Kurz, D. (2005). Men's violence toward women is the serious problem. In D. R. Loseke, R. J. Gelles & M.M. Cavanaugh (Eds.), *Current controversies on family violence* (pp. 79-95). Thousand Oaks, CA: Sage.

Makepeace, J. M. (1986). Gender differences in courtship violence victimization. *Family Relations, 35,* 383-389.

Martin, M. E. (1997). Double your trouble: Dual arrest in family violence. *Journal of Family Violence, 12,* 139-157.

McCarroll, J., Thayer, L., Liu, X., Newby, J., Norwood, A., Fullerton, C., & Ursano, R. (2000). Spouse recidivism in the U.S. Army by gender and military status. *Journal of Consulting and Clinical Psychology, 68,* 521-525.

Mercy, J., & Salzman, L. (1989). Fatal violence among spouses in the United States, 1976-85. *American Journal of Public Health, 79,* 595-599.

Miller, S. L. (2001). The paradox of women arrested for domestic violence: Criminal justice professionals and service providers respond. *Violence Against Women, 7,* 1339-1376.

Miller, S. L., & Meloy, M. L. (2006). Women's use of force: Voices of women arrested for domestic violence. *Violence Against Women, 12*, 89-115.

Moffitt, T. E., & Caspi, A. (1999). *Findings about partner violence from the Dunedin multidisciplinary health and development study.* Washington, DC: National Institute of Justice.

O'Keefe, M. (1998). Posttraumatic stress disorder among incarcerated battered women: A comparison of battered women who killed their abusers and those incarcerated for other offenses. *Journal of Traumatic Stress, 11*, 71-85.

Pence, E., & Paymar, M. (1993). *Education groups for men who batter.* London: Springer.

Peters, J., Shackelford, T., & Buss, D. (2002). Understanding domestic violence against women: Using evolutionary psychology to extend the feminist functional analysis. *Violence and Victims, 17*, 255-265.

Rennison, C. (2003). *Intimate partner violence, 1993-2001.* (Publication No. NCJ197838) Washington, DC: Bureau of Justice Statistics, Department of Justice.

Renzetti, C. (1997). Editor's introduction. *Violence Against Women, 3*, 459-461.

Rodriguez, S. F., & Henderson, V. A. (1993). Intimate homicide: Victim-offender relationship in female perpetrated homicide. *Deviant Behavior: An Interdisciplinary Journal, 16*, 45-57.

Straus, M. A. (1999). The controversy over domestic violence by women: A methological, theoretical and sociology of science analysis. In X. B. Arriaga & S. Oskamp (Eds.) *Violence in intimate relationships* (pp. 17-44). Thousand Oaks, CA: Sage.

Straus, M. A. (2005). Women's violence toward men is a serious social problem. In D. R. Loseke, R. J. Gelles & M. M. Cavanaugh (Eds.), *Current controversies on family violence* (pp. 55-77). Thousand Oaks, CA: Sage.

Straus, M. A., & Gelles, R. J. (1986). Societal change and change in family violence from 1975 to 1985 as revealed by two national surveys. *Journal of Marriage and the Family, 48*, 465-479.

Stovall-McClough, K. C., & Cloitre, M. (2006). Unresolved attachment, PTSD and dissociation in women with childhood abuse histories, *Journal of Counseling and Clinical Psychology, 74*, 219-228.

Stuart, R. (2005). Treatment for partner abuse: Time for a paradigm shift. *Professional Psychology: Research and Practice, 36, 3*, 254-263.

Swan, S., & Snow, D. (2002). A typology of women's use of violence in intimate relationships. *Violence Against Women, 8*, 286-319.

Tjaden, P. G., & Thoennes, N. (1997). *The prevalence and consequences of intimate partner violence: Findings from the National Violence Against Women Survey.* Paper presented at the American Society of Criminology 49th Annual Meeting, San Diego, CA.

van der Hart, O., Nijenhuis, E. R. S., & Steele, K. (2005). Dissociation: An insufficiently recognized major feature of complex posttraumatic stress disorder. *Journal of Traumatic Stress, 18, 5*, 413-423.

Watson, C. (2000). Female perpetrators of domestic violence: A pilot study. (Doctoral Dissertation, United States International University, San Diego, CA, 2000). *Dissertation Abstracts International, 61*, 09B, 5011.

doi:10.1300/J229v08n02_04

Dissociation and Memory for Perpetration Among Convicted Sex Offenders

Kathryn Becker-Blease, PhD
Jennifer J. Freyd, PhD

SUMMARY. Sex abusers' denial of their offenses poses serious problems for their victims, treatment providers, and researchers. Abusers deny their offenses for many reasons, including avoiding responsibility. It is possible that some abusers do not recall their offenses because of intoxication, head injury, or dissociative symptoms that affect their ability to encode or retrieve information. Self-reports of dissociation during childhood victimization, during the perpetration of victimizing acts, and in everyday life were examined in a sample of 17 convicted sex offenders. Half of the participants reported some forgetting of instances when they had sexually abused another person. Forgetting perpetration was related to both dissociation at the time of the offense and dissociation in everyday life. Dissociating while the participants themselves were being physically

Kathryn Becker-Blease is affiliated with Washington State University Vancouver, Psychology Department, VCLS 208U, 14204 NE Salmon Creek Avenue, Vancouver, WA 98686-9600 (E-mail: kblease@vancouver.wsu.edu).

Jennifer J. Freyd is affiliated with the Department of Psychology, 1227 University of Oregon, Eugene, OR 97403-1227 (E-mail: jjf@dynamic.uoregon.edu and jtd@dynamic.uoregon.edu).

This project was funded in part by a graduate student research grant from the Center for the Study of Women in Society at the University of Oregon. Manuscript preparation was supported by the UO Foundation's Fund for Research on Trauma and Oppression.

[Haworth co-indexing entry note]: "Dissociation and Memory for Perpetration Among Convicted Sex Offenders." Becker-Blease, Kathryn, and Jennifer J. Freyd. Co-published simultaneously in *Journal of Trauma & Dissociation* (The Haworth Medical Press, an imprint of The Haworth Press, Inc.) Vol. 8, No. 2, 2007, pp. 69-80; and: *Trauma and Dissociation in Convicted Offenders: Gender, Science, and Treatment Issues* (ed: Kathryn Quina, and Laura S. Brown) The Haworth Medical Press, an imprint of The Haworth Press, Inc., 2007, pp. 69-80. Single or multiple copies of this article are available for a fee from The Haworth Document Delivery Service [1-800-HAWORTH, 9:00 a.m. - 5:00 p.m. (EST). E-mail address: docdelivery@haworthpress.com].

or sexually abused as children was related to both dissociation during later perpetration and everyday dissociation as an adult. The results support continued research and clinical work to determine the frequency of dissociative symptoms and amnesia among sex abusers. doi:10.1300/ J229v08n02_05 *[Article copies available for a fee from The Haworth Document Delivery Service: 1-800- HAWORTH. E-mail address: <docdelivery@haworthpress. com> Website: <http://www.HaworthPress.com> © 2007 by The Haworth Press, Inc. All rights reserved.]*

KEYWORDS. Dissociation, memory, sex offenders, criminal behavior

INTRODUCTION

Sex abusers' denial, minimization, and amnesia for their actions is a serious impediment to holding abusers accountable, validating survivors' experiences, and preventing future abuse. Sex abusers deny their actions for many reasons, including fear of rejection or punishment. Other abusers acknowledge they must have done something, but claim that they cannot remember what they actually did (Hall, 1996; Marshall, Serran, Marshall, & Fernandez, 2005). Although clinicians report a high percentage of clients who intentionally malinger, it is possible that some abusers do not recall their offenses because of intoxication, head injury, or dissociative symptoms that affect their ability to encode or retrieve information (Moskowitz, 2004).

It is difficult to know how frequently abusers claim not to have memory for offenses or how many actually are unable to recall memory for offenses they have committed. Alleged perpetrators of all kinds of crimes claim amnesia (see Moskowitz, 2004 for a review), but these claims, of course, are complicated by a strong motivation to maintain innocence during legal proceedings. Even more problematic is the fact that the majority of sex crimes are never brought to the attention of authorities, making it impossible to know how many offenders claim not to recall offenses when confronted informally, or how many are never confronted with abuse they do not recall. Survivors of childhood sexual abuse frequently report not being believed–a phenomenon in which offender denials may play a significant role (Veldhuis & Freyd, 1999).

In response to the difficulty of treating sex offenders who claim not to remember their offenses, Marshall et al. (2005) published a method for helping convicted sex offenders recover memories of perpetration prior to beginning group treatment. The level of amnesia varied, with most offenders having recall for the day of the abuse, but not the offense itself. Offenders were encouraged to recall repeatedly the events leading up to the offense and events occurring just after until they have recalled details of the offense itself. Presumably the offenders in Marshall et al.'s program were motivated to recover memories, as the only way to enter treatment and qualify for early parole was to first recover the memory. When offenders reported memories of the events, their version was compared with police reports and victim statements to ensure accuracy of the reported memories. Marshall et al. (2005) attempted this technique with 22 convicted male sex offenders, including 10 who said they were intoxicated at the time of the offense and six who claimed to have suffered traumatic head injury. Twenty offenders were able to recover substantially accurate memories of their offenses using this technique. Marshall et al. (2005) did not specifically address dissociation as a possible mechanism of amnesia, and suggest that, at least for treatment, the exact cause of amnesia or whether or not it is feigned may be irrelevant.

The question of whether voluntary perpetration of violence can be viewed as "traumatizing" is controversial (MacNair, 2002; Moskowitz, 2004). Although we do not directly address this controversy here, we are interested in perpetrators' dissociative symptoms in general and at the time they are abusing others. For several reasons, it is likely that sex offenders, as a group, are likely to have dissociative experiences, and that these experiences arise during perpetration.

Trauma History. First, sex offenders, as a group, are a highly traumatized population (Barnard, Hankins, & Robbins, 1992; Simons, Wurtele, & Heil, 2002). Estimates of rates of sexual abuse history among identified adult sex offenders ranges from 25% to 70%, and between 40% and 80% of adolescent sex offenders. A history of child physical abuse has been reported in approximately 50% of sex offenders (see Simons et al., 2002 for a review). A history of child abuse is associated with having dissociative experiences in everyday life, and especially during times of stress (Putnam, 1997). Children who used dissociation to cope with their own victimization may activate the same dissociative cognitive processing style at the time they are perpetrating abuse. The contexts are similar, and some offenders may rely on dissociation to block memories of their own victimization experiences that would otherwise inhibit their own abusive actions. As reviewed by Moskowitz (2004), rates of significant dissociative pathology among sex offenders in non-hospitalized settings range from 9% to 39%.

Fantasy Absorption. Second, sex offenders often report vivid and intense sexual fantasies that lead up to perpetration of victims. Often, these fantasies are supported by the use of pornographic movies, literature, and photographs. The experience of becoming very absorbed in daydreams, fantasies, and movies is a key component of dissociation. For example, the Dissociative Experiences Scale (Bernstein & Putnam, 1986) includes an item that asks how frequently respondents, "find that when you are watching television or a movie you become so absorbed in the story that you are unaware of other events happening around them." Another item asks about times, "you become so involved in a fantasy or daydream that is feels as though it were really happening."

Depersonalization and Derealization. Third, sex offenders frequently objectify their victims, so that they do not view them as real people who feel pain. They sometimes report feeling as though they are watching themselves act from outside their bodies, or as if they are seeing the world in a distorted way (e.g., through a fog). Two related aspects of dissociation (that are also seen in some other psychiatric conditions) could be related to these phenomena for some sex offenders. Derealization is an aspect of dissociation that involves seeing the world as "unreal." Depersonalization is a feeling that one's own self is not real. Derealization and depersonalization are often reported together (Bernstein & Putnam, 1986). A sample DES item is, "Some people sometimes feel as if they are looking at the world through a fog, so that people and objects appear far away or unclear."

Altered Identity. Fourth, it is common for sex offenders to appear to behave quite differently in different contexts. For example, Dennis Radar, convicted of 10 sexually motivated murders, was described this way (Robinson, 2005): "He was a family man, a Cub Scout leader and pastor in his church–all while keeping his double life as the BTK (which stands for 'Bind, Torture, Kill') killer a secret, even from his wife and children." Radar himself referred to his "compartmentalized personalities" (Bardsley, Bell, & Lohr, n.d.). Compartmentalization–"the separation of areas of awareness and memory from each other" (Putnam, 1997, p. 71)–is a major component of dissociation. It is captured by this DES item (Bernstein & Putnam, 1986): "Some people find that in one situation they may act so differently compared with another situation that they feel almost as if they were two different people."

Sex offenders are a diverse group that includes people who have significant psychopathy and who abuse drugs and alcohol. We do not argue that all sex offenders are highly dissociative, but that dissociation is one possible mechanism (separate from or in conjunction with psychopathy and substance abuse) by which offenders are able to ignore, forget, and/ or deny their abuse. For some, dissociation may serve to perpetuate abuse by facilitating intense deviant fantasies, allowing perpetrators to dehumanize their victims, and behave in socially acceptable ways in day-to-day life that make it difficult for society to believe they could be guilty of sex abuse.

In the current study, we were interested in convicted sex offenders' self-reports of their own dissociation symptoms in general, during abuse experienced during childhood, and during perpetration of abuse. We also examined their own appraisals of their memory for their offenses. Specifically, we hypothesized that dissociation during childhood victimization would be related to dissociation during perpetration. In turn, we hypothesized that dissociation during perpetration would be related to memory impairment for perpetration.

METHOD

Participants

Participants were recruited from group therapy sessions at a court-mandated sex offender treatment program. Twenty survey packets were distributed, and seventeen male clients participated. All had been convicted of at least one sex crime against a child or adult. Participants were low income (average annual income = $9060, *SD* = 6068). Age ranged from 26 to 61 years (*m* = 43.3, *SD* = 13.7). Three participants indicated their highest level of education was less than high school. Twelve indicated obtaining a high school diploma or GED. One participant had a 2-year college degree and one had a 4-year degree. Fourteen participants identified as Non-Hispanic White, one as Hispanic white, and two as Native American/White.

Materials

Betrayal Trauma Inventory. Participants completed the physical and sexual abuse items (but not the emotional abuse items) from the Betrayal Trauma Inventory (BTI, Freyd, DePrince, & Zurbriggen, 2001), which assesses detailed information about childhood abuse (prior to age 16). Participants were asked about 34 detailed, behaviorally-defined events. An example physical punishment item asks if "someone punched you with a closed fist, or kicked you, anywhere on your body." A sample childhood sexual experiences asks if "someone had you fondle them (for example, touch or caress their genitals or other parts of their body) in a sexual way."

Abuse-Perpetration Inventory. The perpetration section of the Abuse-Perpetration Inventory (API, Lisak et al., 2000) was used to collect to information about sexual child abuse, adult rape, physical child abuse, and physical violence against an intimate partner. Because the BTI took its initial inspiration from the API, API items are similar to BTI items, in that employ specific, behaviorally-defined descriptions of events. An example item is, "Have you ever performed oral sex on a child close to you?" For all of the questions involving perpetration against a child, questions are repeated for a child "close to you" and "not close to you." Subjects are asked to indicate the number times this event occurred (never, one time, 2-6 times, 6-20 times, 20-100 times, and 100+ times).

Dissociation During Victimization and Perpetration. The 10-item Peritraumatic Dissociation Questionnaire (PDEQ, Marmar, Weiss, & Metzler, 1997) followed each section of the BTI and API. Participants were asked to consider the last time they had any of the experiences they just responded to (e.g., any of the sexual abuse perpetration items) and answer the PDEQ items thinking about their reactions during that experience and immediately after using a 5-point scale. The PDEQ assesses dissociative experiences, such as "I had moments of losing track of what was going on–I "blanked out" or "spaced out" or in some way felt that I was not part of what was going on." PDEQ item scores were averaged, and had a possible range of 1 to 5.

Trait Dissociation. The Dissociative Experiences Scale (DES, Bernstein & Putnam, 1986) is a widely used 28-item self-report survey assessing dissociation in everyday life. Participants rate the amount of times they experienced various experiences, from 0 to 100% of the time (excluding times they were under the influence of drugs or alcohol). A sample item is "Some people have the experience of driving a car and suddenly realizing that they don't remember what has happened during all or part of the trip. Circle a number to show what percentage of the time this happens to you." DES scores have a possible range of 0 to 100. In past research with criminal offenders, scores greater than 30 or 50 have been used to indicate the presence of pathological dissocation.

Social Desirability. The Marlowe-Crowne Social Desirability Scale (Crowne & Marlowe, 1960) is comprised of 32 true-false-items. Questions such as, "Before voting, I always examining the candidates thoroughly before deciding" are asked. Socially desirable responses were coded

"1" and non-socially desirable responses were coded "0," and items were averaged to obtain a mean score.

Memory. Participants were asked four questions about memory for perpetration of sexual abuse. Two questions–"Do you ever find that you've forgotten or blocked out memories about being sexual with a child or unwilling adult?" and "Do thoughts or memories about being sexual with a child or unwilling adult just pop into your head when you are not trying to think about those things?"–used a 5-point response scale from "never" to "almost all the time." Two additional questions– "I think I have totally forgotten about at least one time when I was sexual with a child or unwilling adult" and "I have forgotten about parts or at least one time when I was sexual with a child or unwilling adult"–use a 5-point response scale from "strongly disagree" to "strongly agree."

Procedures

A research assistant announced the opportunity to participate in the study during a group therapy session at a county-funded sexual offender treatment center. The center provides treatment to people convicted of a sexual offense who are mandated to receive treatment during probation or post-prison supervision. Those who consented to participate completed an anonymous survey packet at home and exchanged the completed survey for a $20 gift certificate to a local grocery store. A receptionist at the treatment center accepted the completed packets without disclosing the names of participants to treatment or research staff.

RESULTS

Social Desirability. Social desirability scores ranged from .03 to .83 ($m = 43$. $p = .21$) and were not significantly correlated with state or trait dissociation scores, or any of the memory impairment variables.

Victimization and Perpetration History. Fifteen (88%) participants reported being the victim of childhood physical abuse, including eleven (65%) who reported both child sexual and physical victimization, as assessed by the BTI. No participants reported being the victim of sexual abuse only. Because we did not measure emotional abuse, we do not know the rate of childhood emotional mistreatment in this sample. Six (35%) participants reported sexual abuse perpetration against a child. Eight (47%) participants reported both child and adult victims. Three (18%) participants reported no perpetration, as measured by the API, despite having been convicted of a sex crime. Six (35%) also reported committing physical violence against an intimate partner, and three (18%) also reported physical abuse against a child.

Dissociation During Victimization and Perpetration. Dissociation during child physical or sexual victimization ranged from 1.00 to 3.90 (m = 1.72, SD = .78). Dissociation during perpetration of adult rape or child sex abuse ranged from 1.00 to 3.95 (m = 1.68, SD = 1.02). For the twelve participants who experienced both child physical and/or sexual abuse victimization and who had perpetrated a sex crime against a child and/or adult, the correlation between self-reported dissociation during times being victimized and times perpetrating victimization on another was strong (r = .81, p = 001).

State and Trait Dissociation. DES scores in this sample were highly variable, ranging from 1.43 to 57.86 (m = 16.66, SD = 15.94). Three participants had DES scores greater than 30, including one participant with a score above 50. No scores were more than 3 standard deviations above the mean. DES scores were highly correlated with dissociative experiences reported during child physical and/or sexual abuse victimization (r = .82, p < .001) and perpetration of sex abuse against an adult and/or child (r = .73, p = .005).

Memory for Perpetration. A significant percentage of participants indicated impaired memory for perpetration. Nine (53%) participants said, at least once in awhile, they have "forgotten or blocked out memories about being sexual with a child or unwilling adult." Ten (59%) participants said that, at least once in a while, "thoughts or memories about being sexual with a child or unwilling adult just popped into their heads when they were not trying to think about those things." We did not directly ask if these "thoughts or memories" were of actual abuse the participants had perpetrated. It is possible some participants included times they thought about sexual fantasies or pornography in this figure. Three (18%) participants indicated at least some agreement with the statement, "I think I have totally forgotten about at least one time when I was sexual with a child or unwilling adult." Five (29%) indicated at least some agreement with the statement, "I have forgotten about parts or at least one time when I was sexual with a child or unwilling adult."

Of the three participants who did not admit to any sexual abuse perpetration on the API, two reported that they believed that their memories of abusive behavior were not complete. One said he had "forgotten or blocked out memories about being sexual with a child or unwilling adult" and had "memories about being sexual with a child or unwilling adult just pop into your head when you are not trying to think about those things" once in awhile. The second participant responded "some-times" and "once in awhile" (respectively) to these questions.

The degree to which participants reported they had "forgotten or blocked out memories about being sexual with a child or unwilling adult" was significantly related to both dissociation at the time of perpetration ($r = .79$, $p = .001$) and state dissociation ($r = .73$, $p = .005$).

DISCUSSION

This study is, to our knowledge, the first empirical investigation of both dissociation and memory impairment among convicted sex offenders. Our goal was to investigate possible relations between various forms of dissociation (i.e., during victimization, during perpetration, and in everyday life) and memory impairment for sex offending to determine which of these pathways, if any, merit further systematic research. Our results were consistent with the hypothesis that each of these forms of dissociation and memory impairment are related, and the exact relation indeed does deserve further attention.

Due to variability in samples and measurement methods, previous research does not provide definitive estimates of the rates of childhood abuse and dissociation among sex offenders. However, the rates of sexual abuse and dissociation in the current sample were consistent with the available research. Our rate of physical abuse was somewhat higher than that found in two previous studies.

Dissociation, regardless of type, was highly variable. Some offenders appear to have had very few dissociative experiences, and others experience high levels of dissociation. This finding is consistent with theories of dissociation that suggest that both a predisposition to dissociation, as well as traumatizing event(s) are necessary to produce pathological dissociation (Kluft, 1996).

We hypothesized a relation between dissociation during victimization and dissociation during perpetration. Perhaps some offenders who use dissociation during perpetration first learned to dissociate in order to cope with their own childhood victimization. This could also explain how these offenders manage to ignore their own memories and feelings associated with past abuse during the time they are abusing someone else. Consistent with this hypothesis, we found a strong relation between dissociation during victimization and dissociation during perpetration. Dissociation during victimization and perpetration was also highly related to trait dissociation. Although social desirability scores were not related to any of the dissociation scores, method variance due to other factors may have contributed to the strength of the relation between these measures, which all relied on the same respondent. The magnitude of the correlations, however, suggests that even if a response set bias or other factors were responsible for some of the variance, there is likely some relation between these variables that deserves further research.

Most of the participants reported some memory impairment for sexually abusive events they had perpetrated. This included both not being able to access memories (or parts of memories) as well as intrusive memories. The fact that significant numbers of convicted offenders report memory impairment seems like an extremely important point to consider when evaluating denials by alleged offenders. Popular belief is that sex abuse victimization is so unforgettable and salient that all true victim accounts will be perfectly consistent and complete. Similar logic would suggest offenders should be equally unable to forget sexually abusing another person. The fact that some offenders report the same kinds of memory impairment as victims, even for events they admit they must have committed, opens the door to a more tolerant stance toward both victims' and offenders' accounts for two reasons. First, it adds to the already ample evidence that despite a belief that no one could forget abuse, in fact, people do. Second, it allows us to more fully consider the possibility that a person guilty of sex abuse may provide a seemingly convincing denial because he does not remember doing it. In fact, he may be able to continue appearing to live a model life because memories of his abusive actions are not part of his everyday consciousness. If we were to take this possibility more seriously, we may be more likely to take victims' claims more seriously as well.

Two of the three participants who did not admit to any perpetration on the API reported some memory impairment for abuse. Because of the anonymous nature of the survey, we were unable to follow-up with those participants to find out if they committed a sex crime that was not assessed by the API, if they believed themselves to be wrongly convicted, or if they lacked sufficient memory to report on precisely what abuse they had perpetrated. We plan to directly ask these follow-up questions in future research, and the findings support further inquiry by law enforcement, lawyers, and treatment providers who work with sex offenders who deny perpetrating abuse.

Finally, dissociation during perpetration and in everyday life were related to memory impairment for perpetration. This was not a perfect correlation. Some participants reported memory impairment, but showed low DES scores. This raises the possibility that other factors could be responsible for forgetting (e.g., substance use or head injury) or that the relation between dissociation and memory impairment is more nuanced (e.g., specific dissociative symptoms rather than general dissociation scores are implicated).

This study is limited by factors that have limited other studies of sex offenders. The sample size was small, reflecting the difficulty in identifying and recruiting sex offenders. Nevertheless, strong relations among variables exceeded traditional levels of significance. Sex offenders themselves were the sole reporters for the information obtained. A response set bias could have inflated correlations. Although our social desirability measure was not related to the variables of interest, it is likely offenders' denial and minimization affected their reporting of stigmatizing events. It is difficult to use multi-informant methodologies when the subject of inquiry—internal dissociative processes and secretive crimes—are not visible to observers or reliably measured in other ways. Additional measures of key constructs (e.g., dissociative disorder diagnoses) would strengthen future research on this topic. It will also be important to measure childhood emotional abuse, as recent research suggests such abuse is related to alexithymia (Goldsmith & Freyd, 2005), which could in turn play a role in perpetrator motivation and denial.

Despite these obstacles, this study is the first to indicate a relation between dissociation and memory impairment among convicted sex offenders. This is an important finding that should be explored further because of clear implications for the identification of abuse victims and offenders, for understanding the etiology of sex offending, and for offender treatment.

REFERENCES

Bardsley, M., Bell, R., & Lohr, D. (n.d.). *BTK: Birth of a serial killer.* Retrieved May 26, 2006, from http://www.crimelibrary.com/serial_killers/unsolved/btk/index_1.html.

Barnard, G. W., Hankins, G. C., & Robbins, L. (1992). Prior life trauma, post-traumatic stress symptoms, sexual disorders, and character traits in sex offenders: An exploratory study. *Journal of Traumatic Stress, 5,* 393-420.

Bernstein, E. M., & Putnam, F. W. (1986). Development, reliability, and validity of a dissociation scale. *Journal of Nervous & Mental Disease, 174,* 727-735.

Crowne, D. P., & Marlowe, D. (1960). A new scale of social desirability independent of psychopathology. *Journal of Consulting Psychology, 24,* 349-354.

Freyd, J. J., DePrince, A. P., & Zurbriggen, E. L. (2001). Self-reported memory for abuse depends upon victim-perpetrator relationship. *Journal of Trauma and Dissociation, 2,* 5-17.

Goldsmith, R., & Freyd, J. J. (2005). Awareness for emotional abuse. *Journal of Emotional Abuse, 5,* 95-123.

Hall, G. C. N. (1996). *Theory-based assessment, treatment, and prevention of sexual aggression.* New York: Oxford University Press.

Kluft, R. P. (1996). Dissociative identity disorder. In L. K. Michelson & W. J. Ray (Eds.), *Handbook of dissociation: Theoretical, empirical and clinical perspectives* (pp. 337-366). New York: Plenum Press.

Lisak, D., Conklin, A., Hopper, J., Miller, P., Altschuler, L., & Smith, B. (2000). The Abuse-Perpetration Inventory: Development of an assessment instrument for research on the cycle of violence. *Family Violence & Sexual Assault Bulletin, Spring-Summer,* 21-30.

MacNair, R. M. (2002). *Perpetration-induced traumatic stress.* London: Praeger.

Marmar, C. R., Weiss, D. S., & Metzler, T. J. (1997). The Peritraumatic Dissociative Experiences Questionnaire. In J. P. Wilson & T. M. Keane (Eds.), *Assessing psychological trauma and PTSD* (pp. 412-428). New York: Guilford.

Marshall, W. L., Serran, G., Marshall, L. E., & Fernandez, Y. M. (2005). Recovering memories of the offense in "amnesic" sexual offenders. *Sexual Abuse: A Journal of Research and Treatment, 17,* 31-38.

Moskowitz, A. (2004). Dissociation and violence: A review of the literature. *Trauma, Violence and Abuse, 5,* 21-46.

Putnam, F. W. (1997). *Dissociation in children and adolescents.* New York: Guilford.

Robinson, B. (2005). *Beware the friendly neighborhood killer.* Retrieved May 26, 2006, 2006, from http://abcnews.go.com/US/LegalCenter/story?id=986939&page=1.

Simons, D., Wurtele, S. K., & Heil, P. (2002). Childhood victimization and lack of empathy as predictors of sexual offending against women and children. *Journal of Interpersonal Violence, 17,* 1291-1307.

Veldhuis, C. B., & Freyd, J. J. (1999). Groomed for silence, groomed for betrayal. In M. Rivera (Ed.), *Fragment by fragment: Feminist perspectives on memory and child sexual abuse* (pp. 253-282). Charlottetown, PEI Canada: Gynergy Books.

doi:10.1300/J229v08n02_05

Traumatized Offenders: Don't Look Now, But Your Jail's Also Your Mental Health Center

Philip J. Kinsler, PhD

Anna Saxman, JD

SUMMARY. There are more than a million prison and jail inmates in the United States who have mental illness. As funding for State Hospitals has decreased, funding for needed community programs has often not kept pace. This has led to a population of homeless mentally ill, many of whom have co-occurring substance use disorders. Society's perhaps unconscious response has been to create 24 hour mental health units within prisons and jails. The authors contend that by doing so, we have 're-criminalized' mental illness. The mentally ill prisoner is most often the victim of extreme family turmoil including physical and/or sexual abuse, parental substance dependence, and parental incarceration. Prisons and jails most often do not provide services for this highly traumatized population or recognize the need for such services. The authors report on problematic aspects of mental health care in prisons, and on several attempts to establish 'trauma-aware' care within the legal system. doi:10.1300/J229v08n02_06 *[Article copies available for a fee from The Haworth Document Delivery Service: 1-800-HAWORTH. E-mail address: <docdelivery@haworthpress.com> Website: <http://www. HaworthPress.com>* © 2007 by The Haworth Press, Inc. All rights reserved.]

Philip J. Kinsler is affiliated with Dartmouth Medical School, Hanover, NH.
Anna Saxman is affiliated with the Office of the Defender General, Montpelier, VT.

[Haworth co-indexing entry note]: "Traumatized Offenders: Don't Look Now, But Your Jail's Also Your Mental Health Center." Kinsler, Philip J., and Anna Saxman. Co-published simultaneously in *Journal of Trauma & Dissociation* (The Haworth Medical Press, an imprint of The Haworth Press, Inc.) Vol. 8, No. 2, 2007, pp. 81-95; and: *Trauma and Dissociation in Convicted Offenders: Gender, Science, and Treatment Issues* (ed: Kathryn Quina, and Laura S. Brown) The Haworth Medical Press, an imprint of The Haworth Press, Inc., 2007, pp. 81-95. Single or multiple copies of this article are available for a fee from The Haworth Document Delivery Service [1-800-HAWORTH, 9:00 a.m. - 5:00 p.m. (EST). E-mail address: docdelivery@haworthpress.com].

KEYWORDS. Trauma, mental illness, prisoners, legal system

INTRODUCTION

A staggering total of 1,255,700 persons with serious mental illness are incarcerated in our prison and jail systems (James & Glaze, 2006). How did we get here? In the late 1960's the community psychology movement was launched, in part to help empty out vast warehouses of "mental patients" from State Hospitals that were often inhumane, neglected, decrepit, and cruel. In a few instances, the closing of these hospitals was accompanied with sufficient funding and careful planning for follow-on community programs. In these situations, former psychiatric patients came home to their communities and could live more natural and dignified lives. In far too many cases, the law of unintended consequences applied. Former psychiatric patients were dumped in welfare hotels, farmed out to under funded community agencies–and too often became the core of a homelessness and substance abuse problem in our cities and towns (Stubbs, 1998; Torrey, 1998). The lack of sufficient resources for mental health care in both the public and private sectors has now led to a drastic re-institutionalization of persons with mental illness– in our jails and prisons. Our jails and prisons have become the mental health centers of last resort. We have re-criminalized mental illness.

In September of 2006, the U.S. Department of Justice published the latest in a series of summaries on the mental health problems of incarcerated prisoners. As we have previously noted, the total number of persons "receiving" mental health care in specialized mental health units in prisons and jails is now more than ten times the number of those to be found in State Hospitals (Kinsler & Saxman, 2001). The latest Justice Department report finds that there are some 705,600 persons in State Prisons with mental health problems. This *outnumbers* the number of persons *without* such problems by some 155,700 people. There are 70,200 persons with mental health problems in Federal prisons, and 479,900 such persons in local jails.

Looked at on a percentage basis, we see the following:

- 56.2% of State prison inmates have diagnosable mental health problems.
- 44.8% of Federal prisoners have mental health problems.
- 64.2% of local jail inmates have mental health problems.

- 32% of all incarcerated prisoners show symptoms of Major Depressive Disorder. Twenty-eight percent of inmates show symptoms of Mania. Some 16% show symptoms of Psychosis including hallucinations and delusions.
- "Three quarters of female inmates in State prisons who had a mental health problem met criteria for substance dependence or abuse" (James & Glaze, 2006, p. 10); some 40% of prisoners of both genders who had mental health problems had a co-occurring substance abuse disorder.

Our jails and prisons, in particular our local jails, have become *the* institutional repository for the mentally ill in our communities. These statistics do not simply arise from asking prisoners whether they have any problems. They are the result of careful multi-stage sampling and personal interviewing conducted by the Department of Justice (described in James & Glaze, 2006).

We know from various national studies (as cited in other papers in this volume and in Harlow, 1999) that a substantial proportion of incarcerated offenders report having been sexually abused in childhood. "State prisoners who had a mental health problem were over two times more likely than those without (10%) to report being physically or sexually abused in the past" (James & Glaze 2006, p. 5).

In addition, some 52% of the prisoners with mental health problems grew up in a home where one or both of the *parents* had been incarcerated. Prisoners with mental health problems grew up in families with double the rates of *parental* alcoholism or substance abuse as those without mental health diagnoses. We previously coined a tongue-in-cheek syndrome to describe the lives of large numbers of people who are in prison–we said they suffer from 'horrible life disorder' (Kinsler & Saxman, 2001).

We have been gathering some data on Vermont criminal defendants who come through the Office of the Defender General, which is the public defense arm of Vermont state government. We have statistics on a four-county sample gathered while we had a Department of Justice Grant to aid mentally challenged (e.g., low IQ) defendants, covering a two year period; and from a single county over the same two year period and the subsequent two years.

Table 1 shows that Vermont in many ways tracks the national statistics. Almost 54% of those seen at arraignment have been in mental health treatment previously. Statistics for those in special education

TABLE 1

VT Statistics	Number	Percentage
Total Screened–4 Counties	1081	
Prior Mental Health Treatment	582	53.84%
Clients with IEP's or Special Ed History	195	18.04%
Windham County–Four Years of Data		
Total Screened–Windham County	504	
Prior Mental Health Treatment	333	66.07%
Clients with IEP's or Special Ed History	51	10.12%

Note: Windham County is by Vermont standards an urban county containing a mid-size city and suburbs.

range from about 10-20%. Vermont public defenders are seeing a population with highly significant mental health and educational disabilities.

In summary, large numbers of persons in prison have serious mental health problems, and substantial proportions of these prisoners have been physically or sexually abused, with the proportional risk substantially higher for women.

It can be argued that we are incarcerating people who cope with their own prior abuse through three common pathways; depression, anger and violence, and substance abuse. In many ways, we are incarcerating last generation's abuse survivors, rather than treating them.

On a personal level, this can be shocking, startling, and mind-altering. One goes into work in prisons and jails after receiving an incessant bombardment by the culture about being 'tough on crime.' Presidential campaigns are won and lost on this battleground. Yet, the more time one spends in prisons, the more one sees inmates as victims, abuse survivors, people who never had a chance ... in other words, people very much like our other therapy clients. One walks in with prejudices and comes out with compassion.

THE DELIVERY OF MENTAL HEALTH SERVICES IN JAILS AND PRISONS

The authors have extensive experience in the jail and prison systems in Vermont and New Hampshire. In these states, we have encountered the following kinds of problems in serving the significant numbers of mentally ill inmates within these systems:

- In county jails within New Hampshire, there is rarely any full time medical or mental health staff. Medical services are provided by contracted physicians on a part-time basis. If there are any mental health services they are contracted out on a very limited basis. Jails often do not allow even AA or NA meetings to prisoners who have not yet pled or been sentenced.
- Vermont has an integrated prison system in which regional institutions house all prisoners, both those awaiting adjudication and those already sentenced. In this system, there is full-time medical care. Prescriptions are dispensed by nurse-practitioners to inmates with psychological symptoms, under the part-time supervision of a psychiatrist. Often to cut costs, inmates are prescribed 'last generation' medications such as tricyclics for depression, rather than the more current SSRI's.
- There is one Vermont facility that contains a 24-hour mental health ward. Male prisoners with significant mental health problems are transferred here. Staffing is short. Most 'services' consist of brief suicidality checks and medication management. There is virtually no therapy provided, other than a weekly 15-minute session with a clinician. But the situation is better in the women's prisons. In one of the prisons, called Dale, there is a mental health unit which does provide some treatment.
- It is virtually impossible for an outside therapist to maintain therapeutic contact with their patient once they are housed in a jail or prison, in either state. All service delivery is under the aegis of the Departments of Corrections who are often concerned primarily with liability protection. Dr. Kinsler's offers to provide pro-bono trauma treatment to certain actively PTSD prisoners have been refused.
- Attempts to organize trauma-aware services throughout the Vermont prison system have been unsuccessful, particularly where male prisoners are concerned. The responsible official refused to consider this because it might "open up" prisoners' past conflicts which they would then act out. Department of Corrections officials have been unwilling to see the actively PTSD inmates who are either acting against themselves via self-mutilation or against the staff through rebellion precisely *because* their trauma is not being attended to.
- Well-meaning mental health staffs of the Departments of Corrections are too overburdened to provide extensive care.
- Sometimes, mental health providers 'rise through the ranks' of Corrections Officers and provide 'programming' of a therapeutic nature with no specific psychologically-based training.

- Trauma-based symptoms such as dissociation, psychic numbing, and flashbacks are often seen as lack of cooperation and lead to prisoners being 'failed' at their treatment. Discussing past trauma is often seen as engaging in prohibited self pity or taking a victim role. Having a flashback to a trauma during anger management treatment, for example, can result in a prisoner being judged as disruptive, dismissed from the program, and reported as non-cooperative to the judge.
- The therapies offered in prison often include exercises such as journaling of thoughts and feelings which may provoke trauma-based reactions in the inmate population, and/or may be impossible for them to perform due to low cognitive capacity and learning disabilities. Again, failure to complete these assignments is seen as lack of cooperation with the rehabilitation program.
- The types of treatments offered in jails and prisons are often not empirically validated and of dubious value. The controversy over the effectiveness of sex-offender treatment is beyond the scope of this article. For a cogent discussion of the utility of so-called anger management programs see "Is Anger a Thing-To-Be-Managed?" (Roffman, 2004).
- Even if the programs are of value, there are far fewer "seats" available in the programs than inmates who need the programs. This can lead to often arbitrary policies such as not offering sex-offender treatment to "low-risk" offenders, despite the high error rate of such prediction instruments (Quinsey, Harris, Rice, & Cormier, 2000).
- Finally, and most obviously, prisons are traumatizing places. They are loud. Doors slam with a strident, startling metallic clang. Guards and other prisoners sometimes bellow. Bodily fluids are sometimes flung through cell bars. Most importantly, common expectations of humane treatment of one human being towards another often do not apply. So, our jails and prisons take in already traumatized individuals and place them in re-traumatizing environments. For a rather startling view of life in prison, see *You Got Nothing Coming: Notes of a Prison Fish* (Lerner, 2003).

ILLUSTRATIVE CASE EXAMPLES

Here are two cases from the senior author's forensic work that illustrate some of the issues discussed above, and also demonstrate what we observe to be rather paradigmatic pathways to prison for men and women.

JJ–An Exceptional Athlete–and Hidden Sexual Abuse Survivor– A Common Male Path to Prison

The senior author was brought in to evaluate JJ, who appeared to be decompensating in prison while awaiting trial on alleged kidnapping and sexual assault charges. He was accused of burglary and assaulting a woman physically and sexually. In jail, he was having crying jags, made attempts to hang himself with a sheet, and told his lawyer that he couldn't sleep because of the "nightmares." His attorney and the prison authorities were concerned about possible suicide risk. Suicide attempts or threats in jail are not seen by corrections staff, including some correctional mental health staff, as reflecting emotional disturbance. They are often viewed as a form of misbehavior for which corrections officers, doctors, and supervisors can get in trouble. Therefore, suicidal behaviors often lead to an inmate's placement in an isolation/observation cell, sometimes naked, and sometimes in a "suicide smock:" essentially a straightjacket that prevents a person from using their hands to do themselves harm. Such an intervention satisfies the corrections system's need to control a prisoner, but is ineffective and even potentially dangerous as a response to actual suicidality.

JJ avoided this form of abusive intervention in large part because he was locally famous as a former star football player for his high school team. I (PK) was asked to perform a consult. JJ's public defender did a wonderful job convincing JJ that it was safe to talk to me, that I would listen. I taped the sessions for reasons of self-protection and later evidentiary use if necessary, a common practice in forensic psychology. Asking JJ about his family during a simple history-taking broke the dam. He was sobbing so wretchedly I couldn't follow the words. He was gasping for breath. He was tearing at his hair and face. He told me that he'd never shared any of this with anyone before because it wasn't manly and no one would care anyway. His story was that he was one of six children born to the town bully. The bully was determined that each one of his sons would also be, no matter what the price. JJ described hours of 'practices' where Dad would beat him with a cow harness if he didn't perform correctly. Dad's rages were legendary, and no one bucked him. Not surprisingly, one of JJ's uncles also became a sadist–and enjoyed turning this on JJ, the littlest child. This uncle proceeded to anally rape JJ whenever they were left alone. He later sold JJ to his friends for similar use. JJ started using alcohol and drugs for self-soothing as soon as he was able, well before the age of 10. As an adolescent he gravitated towards extremely dysfunctional women with similar family backgrounds and drug habits.

Despite his past, he stoutly denied any sexual contact with the woman whose house he burgled, and the DNA evidence excluded him.

Psychological trauma survivors attempt to cope with and 'master' their traumatic experiences in a variety of ways that re-enact some part of their traumatic experience. They may unconsciously choose partners who will mistreat them in similar ways to their abusive experiences. This is done to try to 're-write the ending' of the trauma–"Maybe I can succeed in making them love me *this time*." They may also 'identify with the aggressor' and try to re-establish a sense of competency and power by acting towards others in the ways they were acted upon. They may become repeatedly masochistic, their repeated victimization 'proving' to them that the world really is just … "These things happen to me because I am a terrible person." This can allow them to preserve the illusion that if they were 'better' their parents would have treated them with love. Quite often, survivors unconsciously adopt several of these strategies as they attempt to cope with current 'triggers' in their lives (Van der Kolk, 1989).

JJ's actions can be viewed productively through several different trauma-informed lenses. JJ felt powerless and terrified, as he did as a child. He acted as the powerful figures in his childhood had acted. He attempted to master his powerlessness by mimicking how his abusers had treated him. Having been bullied, held down, and restrained, when his terror was aroused, he did this to someone else.

A second productive view is to conceptualize JJ as a person with borderline personality disorder about to lose a love object. He shows the hyper-vigilance and hyper-reactivity to relationship loss of someone who has been multiply traumatized and terrorized. His behaviors are reminiscent of what Stosny has called Attachment Abuse–how abused men sometimes act when the bottom drops out of attachments they depend on (Stosny 1995, 2004). As the terror of being alone and bereft of safety increases, the person's desperate clinging to the loved object increases, sometimes leading to restraint and confinement types of abusive acts.

Neither of these lenses has been used to conceptualize JJ's case. After a plea agreement, he is serving time with minimal or no mental health services. If and when he is released, the core problems of a traumatized man who can act out under threat of loss will still remain. He will still be in tremendous pain, and society will be in no less danger.

BC, a Common Female Path to Prison

BC, hereinafter known as Brandi, grew up on a traditional Vermont farm and was used to working the 7 day a week, first-light to darkness schedule of the dairy farmer. Her father died in his 40's and Brandi and her brother took over running the place and caring for their mother. Brandi was not interested in typical 'female' things but in horses, cows, four-wheelers, and fishing. And so, she was something of a social outcast. After her father's death she paid little attention to school even though an older brother was attending college. Every minute away from the farm was a minute wasted to her; there were chores that had to be done. Her father had 'worked out' at different jobs to supplement the family's income. Brandi did the same. In keeping with her father's wishes, she did barely complete high school. We enter the story of Brandi's life after high school graduation when her self-esteem and choice of partners leads her to alcohol, criminal behavior, and eventually jail.

After high school, Brandi worked for a manufacturing company. Her co-workers had lunch at a bar across the street; they would drink, play pool, and then go back to work. She had her first drink there. She had a friend who was one year younger; when that friend reached legal age they would 'start hitting the bars.' Her drinking was 'social' and was 'fine.' It had not reached the problematic level. She would drink on weekends at a certain bar, and moved to another when the first went out of business. At this second bar she met Tony and 'stayed with him for a while.' He 'managed to leave her pregnant and bewildered.' She had an abortion … 'Not ready to raise a kid, still raising me.'

She then met Billy, a truck driver, whom she married. It was an abusive relationship. She went out on the road driving truck with him. It became a classic control story. He would prevent her from keeping in contact with her mother, looming over her when she tried to phone home. He would hit her; he knocked her down by hitting her with the door of the truck. He would 'hit her if she put her arm in the wrong place' in the truck. She 'became his punching bag.' He would 'take trips, like to Kentucky, so she couldn't get away from him and go home.' She told her brother 'Mikey' what was going on. Mike then 'drove through a huge storm to come get her.' She managed to leave Billy for a time, then 'thought she could fix things' and 'went back out [on the road] with him for a while.' The abuse and beating continued. Billy continued the pattern of taking loads where Brandi could not get back to New England. She was finally able to gather the courage to call her grandmother and to demand that Billy leave while the phone line was open so her grandmother could hear. He complied and left, and they were divorced in a local County Court. Billy 'did not show up, didn't pay off the credit cards–she had even charged the wedding rings.' This last statement is something of a metaphor for her relationships with men. *She chooses men she describes as 'losers' and then tries to prove her worth to them by doing everything for them.* She is always the out-cast trying to be taken in.

The pattern repeated a year later when she met Louie. He was a man 28 years her senior. She spent '8 years of wasted time' with Louie. She 'thought he would be the one who would take care of her.' They shared interests in 'hunting, fishing, motorcycles, deer camp.' Then it turned in to 'everything she did [was] not good enough' for him. The 'more she tried to do, the more he would tell you he could do better … take care of him like a complete baby … cut his firewood … put it in … anything he said … not good enough … [he made me] feel like I was useless.' He was continually verbally abusive and in particular tried to attack any sense of worth, in order to establish total power over Brandi. She had stopped any drinking for more than a year. He would 'drink in front of her, keep offering it to her.' There was an active pattern of trying to sub-vert any sense of self-confidence or competence. Reality was twisted until she was to blame for everything, and she began to believe this. She gave me an example of Louie's truck. At one point, he became an-gry and essentially destroyed the tailgate of this truck in a rage, when he had trouble opening it. He then blamed her for not properly oiling the hinges. She was doing all his car maintenance, but whatever she did was not right. She believed she was at fault for not taking better care of the hinges.

He would try to prevent her from seeing her mother, who was elderly and sick. He tried to keep her from contact with Mike. It was a classic power and control relationship, with Brandi continually put down and subject to constant verbal abuse. He accused her of a lesbian relation-ship with her sister Sally and her best friend Rita. He accused her of sleeping with her brother Mikey. In her excellent words 'he kept upping the degradation.' She felt that she had to 'protect the family' from what was happening to her; she was ashamed and also felt that if Mikey knew he would 'go ballistic' at Louie.

Brandi reports that she tried to leave Louie and that when she did so 'he tried to put her mother in a ditch' while driving. She became afraid of what he would do to her family if she stayed apart from him, and so went back to him. She had resumed drinking and was drinking a lot at this point. She was 'no help in the barn' to her family.

For a time, she was able to preserve some self-esteem, and her own independent perception of what was going on between her and Louis, because she was working at a furniture company. However, she hurt her back and had to be off work. Louie thought this meant 'she could sit home and do his bidding.' 'As long as she was home, she could do everything for him.' There's 'no way to explain, you have to be there.' At one point, she had a broken leg. After three days he was verbally attacking her for not doing the work around the place ... 'Why can't you walk on it?'

When a person lives with constant abuse, their sense of themselves and their reality changes. Brandi felt 'she was never going to amount to anything–he was so much like me–hunting, fishing ... if I can't please him how can I please anyone ... everything my fault ... if I'da done that he wouldn't have smashed the tail gate.' The abused person lives in a reality in which they cannot see clearly; they are the awful ones, the shameful ones, the ones responsible for what is happening to them.

To cope with these feelings, Brandi was drinking and using the pain pills from her back. She 'knew she wanted to leave for the better part of a year.' She did 'not know how to do it without Louie endangering the family–to make her come back.' She 'gotta find a way to get away from him.' At first she would 'ride around on back roads to figure out a way to do it. For a while just drink, drive, fish ... make it worse 'cause things not done to home.'

At one point, she was at a fishing hole. She 'saw a camp ... wondered what was inside.' She went inside and 'smashed the place up a little bit and left.' When I asked her to reflect on what she was feeling at the time, she replied that she was 'pretending it was his stuff ... smashing to hell ... but so drunk not remember a lot of it.' This smashing incident occurred before the first fire or shooting incident by her report. She 'just left.' She became 'paranoid' that somebody would find out it was her. She says she decided to 'go back, use fire, destroy evidence ... burn it down.'

At this point, I asked her about fires that by my records had occurred during an earlier period; she thought a while and then told me that she 'shot up the local rod and gun club' and some other hunting camps. There was 'no reason for it–not mad at anyone in those camps.' It appeared to be a way of her expressing all the anger she was carrying around from her relationship with Louie, to this examiner. When talking about this, Brandi was very ashamed, holding her stomach and almost doubled over with shame. She thought that the first fire was 'just gonna take care of it and forget about it … but it didn't stop is all.' She 'thought she could leave it alone.' She 'doesn't remember where the second one was.' She connects her setting fires to times when she and Louie would get in arguments. They had a fight when she asked him to help pay her car insurance. She had been doing everything around the house and repairing all his vehicles. He responded 'Why should I take care of your bills?' Brandi says that she set fires 'to get back at him … make the fire department look bad … he was on the fire department 30 years.'

In this example, we see a woman made powerless and self-hating, who re-enacts this by being demeaning and destructive to others. In this case, thank goodness, there are no visible, personal victims, but instead Brandi harms property with the same kind of rage that she has been so often been subjected to. In common with many other female victims, she has also turned to substance abuse, likely as a way to disinhibit her own prohibitions about expressing anger.

And in common with the prior example of JJ, she is now serving a long sentence for arson with very limited mental health services. Therefore, she may again choose someone demeaning and abusive as her next partner, increasing her already intolerable level of personal pain; and also once again putting the community at risk that she will re-offend.

Brandi's story cannot, of course, capture all the complex reasons why women find themselves in abusive relationships, and the difficulties they experience in attempting to leave these, in a society with often minimal supports for abused women. For a fuller theoretical discussion of these issues, see the work of Angela Browne (Browne, 1991; 1993).

ATTEMPTS TO PROVIDE SERVICES TO THE MENTALLY ILL AND/OR DEVELOPMENTALLY DELAYED POPULATION

In recognition of some of the factors discussed above, the authors initially attempted to develop a program of aid and support in court hearings for defendants of low IQ who had still been judged competent to stand trial. This appeared the most politically obtainable goal; various stake-holders all agreed that it would be a good idea to provide services to defendants who could barely understand what was going on in the courtroom–and prosecutors agreed that these very same people were seen as victims as often as they were as perpetrators. The developmentally delayed person could as easily come to the court's attention as a victim of domestic violence as they could for resisting arrest or simple assault on a police officer, for example. We have reported this project in detail in a previous article (Kinsler & Saxman, 2001).

We envisioned a project that would provide support and aid to the defendants. While we were successful in eventually raising the attorneys' awareness of the limitations of many of their clients, and we offered creative solutions for many clients with limitations, there were some negative results concerning the use of "cognitive facilitators" or communication support persons. These persons were trained to help assist the developmentally disabled defendants whose understanding of the court process or legal documents was marginal, at best. Some prosecutors and state examiners, however, used the program to "push marginally competent subjects over the line." In other words, persons who might have been judged as incompetent to stand trial, and therefore have their cases dismissed or referred to a hospital, were now being judged competent to go forward in the legal system because they could have the support of the cognitive facilitators provided by the program. The program was being used to "make the incompetent, competent." Attorneys involved with the program came to believe it was being used *against* the clients' interests. In fact, they resented making referrals to the program and did not wish to cooperate with it. The program was terminated based upon a loss of grant funding and the reaction from the Public Defender attorneys, although a smaller version provides cognitive facilitators in Family Court, where helping mentally ill persons show themselves as competent with some social support can work in the client's best interests.

We have made other attempts to introduce support services and trauma-focused treatment in the Vermont Corrections system. However, analysis of a request for proposal from the State of Vermont to contract to provide mental health services in Vermont prisons required providing very limited services or dramatically under-paying the providers and generating excessive staff turnover. The senior author's academic department declined to bid under these circumstances.

Another challenge we encountered from a former Clinical Director of the Corrections Department who stated that they did not want to "open up" issues leading to prisoners becoming actively PTSD and therefore vulnerable to other prisoners. The fact that the prisoners already had active PTSD, and that they were acting out their issues continually within the prison system, did not make an impact on the system or lead to openness to trauma services. This experience is consistent with that described by other authors attempting to address trauma in corrections systems (Browne, 1991; Browne, Miller, & Magulin, 1999).

Finally, the senior author continues to provide "subtle" trauma treatment services within an informal network which includes trauma-sensitive attorneys and individual personnel within the system. While this informal system aids in some cases, it is far from the encompassing approach to traumatized offenders we would like to see.

We do see some progress, however. One county, Chittenden County, which is where Burlington, Vermont's largest city and the University of Vermont are located, has recently begun a mental health court for mentally ill offenders charged with repeated misdemeanors. No statistics are currently available to judge the success of this experiment or to compare it to a similar county without such a court. The authors hope to track progress and gather data in the future.

In conclusion, in prisons and jails we see deeply wounded and highly traumatized persons, who are placed in a highly traumatizing situation, with little to no trauma-aware care and limited political openness to providing this.

REFERENCES

Browne, A. (1991). The victim's experience: Pathways to disclosure. *Psychotherapy, 28*(1), 150-156.

Browne, A. (1993). Violence against women by male partners: Prevalence, outcomes and policy implications. *American Psychologist, 48*(10), 1077-1087.

Browne, A., Miller, B., & Margulin, E. (1999). Prevalence and severity of lifetime physical and sexual victimization among incarcerated women. *International Journal of Law & Psychiatry, 22*(3-4), 301-322.

Harlow, C. (1999). Prior abuse reported by inmates and probationers [NCH 172879]. Bureau of Justice Statistics, April.

James, D., & Glaze, L. (2006). Mental health problems of prison and jail inmates [NCJ 213600]. Office of Justice Programs, September.

Kinsler, P., Saxman, A., & Fishman, D. (2004). The Vermont defendant accommodation project: A case study. *Psychology, Public Policy, and Law, 10*(1-2), 134-161.

Lerner, J. (2003). *You got nothing coming: Notes of a prison fish.* New York: Broadway Books.

Quinsey, V., Harris, G., Rice, M., & Cormier, C. (1998). *Violent offenders: Appraising and managing risk.* Washington, DC: American Psychological Association.

Roffman, A. (2004). Is anger a thing-to-be-managed? *Psychotherapy: Theory, Research, Practice, Training, 41*(2), 161-171.

Stosny, S. (1995). *Treating attachment abuse: A compassionate approach.* New York: Springer.

Stosny, S. (2004). *Manual of the Core Value Workshop.* Charleston, SC: Booksurge Publishing.

Stubbs, P. (1998). Broken promises: The story of deinstitutionalization. [Online]. *Perspectives, 3*(4). Retrieved October 30, 2006 from www.mentalhelp.net/poc/view_doc.php? type=doc&id=368

Torrey, E. (1998). *Nowhere to go–The tragic odyssey of the homeless mentally ill*. New York: Harper & Row.

Van der Kolk, B. (1989). The compulsion to repeat the trauma: Re-enactment, revictimization and masochism. *Psychiatric Clinics of North America, 12*(2), June, 389-411.

doi:10.1300/J229v08n02_06

Developing and Assessing Effectiveness of a Time-Limited Therapy Group for Incarcerated Women Survivors of Childhood Sexual Abuse

Kimberly L. Cole, PsyD
Pamela Sarlund-Heinrich, PsyD
Laura S. Brown, PhD

SUMMARY. A thorough search of the literature has revealed little empirical research on the effects of trauma therapy with incarcerated women with histories of CSA. Psychotherapy, when available in a correctional setting, seems more related to resolving immediate crises that interfere with smooth management of the corrections environment rather than dealing with underlying problems such as CSA. The purpose of this preliminary investigation therefore was to implement and evaluate the efficacy of a time-limited, trauma-focused group intervention with a group of recently-incarcerated women volunteers who had experienced

Kimberly L. Cole and Pamela Sarlund-Heinrich are affiliated with Greater Lakes Mental Healthcare, Lakewood, WA.

Laura S. Brown is Director, Fremont Community Therapy Project, Seattle, WA.

The authors wish to thank John Haroian, PhD, without whom this study would not have been possible.

[Haworth co-indexing entry note]: "Developing and Assessing Effectiveness of a Time-Limited Therapy Group for Incarcerated Women Survivors of Childhood Sexual Abuse." Cole, Kimberly L., Pamela Sarlund-Heinrich, and Laura S. Brown. Co-published simultaneously in *Journal of Trauma & Dissociation* (The Haworth Medical Press, an imprint of The Haworth Press, Inc.) Vol. 8, No. 2, 2007, pp. 97-121; and: *Trauma and Dissociation in Convicted Offenders: Gender, Science, and Treatment Issues* (ed: Kathryn Quina, and Laura S. Brown) The Haworth Medical Press, an imprint of The Haworth Press, Inc., 2007, pp. 97-121. Single or multiple copies of this article are available for a fee from The Haworth Document Delivery Service [1-800-HAWORTH, 9:00 a.m. - 5:00 p.m. (EST). E-mail address: docdelivery@haworth press.com].

Available online at http://jtd.haworthpress.com

doi:10.1300/J229v08n02_07

CSA. Five women completed the group plus pre- and post-test measures; a wait-list control group completed measures at the same intervals. Results were mixed in regard to the effectiveness of treatment: decreases were found in the mean Trauma Content (TC/R) scores of the Rorschach Inkblot Method (RIM), but scores on the TSI and the SCL-90-R did not vary greatly. However, women in the control group showed consistent declines in scores during the wait-list period, suggesting the intervention may have helped newly incarcerated women adjust with less symptomatology. doi:10.1300/J229v08n02_07 *[Article copies available for a fee from The Haworth Document Delivery Service: 1-800- HAWORTH. E-mail address: <docdelivery@haworthpress.com> Website: <http://www. HaworthPress.com>* © *2007 by The Haworth Press, Inc. All rights reserved.]*

KEYWORDS. Child sexual abuse, incarcerated women, psychotherapy

INTRODUCTION

Unaddressed consequences of child sexual abuse (CSA), especially repetitive abuse at the hands of a trusted caregiver, may include the development of PTSD, complex PTSD, depression, eating disorders, anxiety disorders, substance abuse disorders, sexual disorders, dissociative disorders, self-mutilation and suicidality. CSA can disrupt or impair developmental tasks, personality development and/or affect regulation, leading to a shortage of healthy coping strategies. As a result, any or all of the preceding disorders may in fact be methods of "coping," used to alleviate the distress from the original trauma (Bloom; 1997; Courtois, 2004; 1997; Elmone & Lingg, 1996; Robinson, 2000). Elmone and Lingg report that their belief is when treating women survivors it is useful to conceptualize these disorders as the aftereffects of sexual abuse, although clearly other risk factors may be implicated in a specific woman's constellation of symptoms. To provide efficacious treatment for the overt symptoms presented by a survivor, the original trauma of CSA must be directly addressed and worked through.

These consequences also include an increased likelihood of becoming a criminal defendant as well as an increased risk of recidivism by CSA survivors with a prior history of incarceration. Female inmates pose a different set of challenges to prison systems, as they have higher rates of psychological problems in comparison to men. These include such issues as Posttraumatic Stress Disorder (PTSD), drug and alcohol abuse, self- and other-injury, and depression. For example, according to Browne, Miller, and Maguin (1999), a substantial majority of women in correctional facilities report having experienced sexual molestation and/or severe physical violence at the hands of others prior to their incarceration, frequently resulting in the multi-faceted symptom picture of complex trauma (Herman, 1992). In a one-year study conducted by Browne et al., of 150 women incarcerated six years or longer at Bedford Hills Maximum Security Corrections Facility (BHCF) in New York, 70% had experienced severe childhood physical violence and 59% reported experiencing some form of sexual abuse during childhood or adolescence. Unfortunately, physical and sexual abuse often continued into adulthood for approximately 75% of the responding women in these studies in the form of severe physical abuse and/or marital sexual assault or exploitation by intimate partners (Bradley & Davino, 2002). If, in fact, we consider the utilization of drugs or alcohol to numb the painful affects associated with repeated interpersonal violence a type of dissociative coping strategy, then the presence of so much such trauma in the lives of women offenders should not be a surprise.

A review of statistics from the Washington State Department of Corrections (DOC; 2005) supports this national trend regarding CSA histories in incarcerated women and confirms its presence in Washington State. All women entering the prison system in Washington come through WCCW after conviction, with many serving out their entire sentences at this all-female facility. The most recent statistics gathered on the WCCW population reveal the following: of the 555 offenders entering prison in a three month period in 2005, 67% had a DSM-IV-TR Axis I diagnosis, 85% met the criteria for chemical dependence, and 32% had a history of at least one suicidal gesture. Additionally, many of the incoming offenders reported that they had experienced some form of abuse, including CSA, childhood physical abuse, rape, and/or domestic violence. Specifically, 46% of the female offenders reported at intake that they had experienced CSA: of these 72% were also physically abused as children, 58% had been raped as an adult, and 79% of these women had also been in a domestically violent relationship (Walker, 2005). All of these experiences are implicated in the development of a complex trauma picture and the presence of dissociative symptoms, which in turn can both increase risk for criminal incarceration and increase risk of recidivism. The overwhelming majority of these incarcerated women entering WCCW had drug-related charges (John Haroian, PhD, personal communication, October 5, 2005). As these are self-reports to correctional staff, the actual numbers may be higher than reported, with some offenders either dissociating knowledge of childhood trauma or not choosing to report it at the time of their incarceration.

Similar statistics regarding women offenders' histories of childhood and adult physical and sexual abuse came to light in the late 1980's during the course of litigation by women residents at WCCW against the Department of Corrections (Jordan v. Gardner, 986 F.2d 1521, 9th Cir., 1993), suggesting that this is a consistent and historical trend rather than a recent or unique development.

Thus, the potential for a history of CSA among incarcerated women is an issue that deserves attention. CSA can affect an individual's perspectives of self and others, leading to long-term interpersonal and intrapersonal consequences in the form of symptoms of distress and problematic and dysfunctional behaviors (Briere, 1992). Considering the multiple impacts of CSA may ultimately provide a useful strategy for clinicians attempting to understand the complex nature of the problems and symptoms present in the female prison population. These consequences may not fit neatly within the confines of those DSM-IV-TR diagnoses that are officially recognized as more serious and trauma-linked in nature. For example, complex trauma is not always accompanied by frank symptoms of PTSD or Dissociative Identity Disorder (DID), as some of the dissociative coping strategies used by women in the penal system involve substance abuse as well as more typically recognized forms of dissociation. However, the current system of prison mental health care delivery is based on DMS-IV-TR categories. In spite of deeply impaired capacities to function due to a range of post-traumatic and dissociative elements, some female offenders are not eligible for routine mental health services under either state or federal mandates regarding mental health services to offender populations. Compounding this is the rationing of all mental health services, a consequence of flat funding at a time of increased prison populations. As a result, at Washington Correction Center for Women (WCCW), as is true at many prisons, individual psychotherapy is a luxury, and group therapies are usually focused on specific coping skills or targeted to behaviors which were prominent in the offenses leading to conviction, such as anger dysregulation or alcohol/drug abuse. The incarcerated female who experiences terror when touched by a man, who "spaces out," or who engages in trauma re-enactments both with other women and with men on the outside, is unlikely to receive treatment targeted at her post-traumatic survival skills, unless those survival skills were implicated in her charged offense or have led to an identifiable serious mental illness.

According to Covington (1998) and the National Institute of Justice (NIJ; 1998), the unique needs of women in prison settings are quite different from those of men, in large part due to women's disproportionate histories of physical and/or sexual victimization. More than 43% of women in prisons (compared to 12% of men) reported physical and/or sexual abuse histories prior to their incarceration. Due to higher rates of exposure to this set of risk factors, women offenders are more likely than men to have drug and/or alcohol problems and mental illnesses, and to have been unemployed prior to incarceration, even taking gender differences in employment rates into account (NIJ, 1998). Compared to their male counterparts women in prison used more drugs and in greater quantities prior to incarceration (Bureau of Justice Statistics, 2000). Again, this points to the use of a chemically enhanced dissociative coping strategy in women who end up in the criminal justice system.

In recent years, incarcerated women have become the focus of considerable research. Researchers have set out to gain insight into the lives of this rapidly growing and all too often forgotten population. It is useful to grasp the enormity of the post-traumatic picture that they present in understanding why the present authors deemed it so important to investigate trauma-focused treatments for such women. In every aspect of their lives, most women who live some parts of their adult lives in prison are at the end point of a trajectory that began with childhood maltreatment, frequently including childhood sexual abuse, which was the focus of our study. The majority of female offenders come from impoverished backgrounds, are poorly educated, have limited access to healthcare resources and have long-standing mental and emotional difficulties as well as long histories of substance abuse (Bureau of Justice Statistics, 2000; Covington, 2003; Maeve, 2000).

It is estimated that 70 to 80% of all incarcerated women are single mothers of young children (Bureau of Justice Statistics, 2000). Many of these women had children as adolescents, a common sequel of childhood sexual abuse. When they are imprisoned those children are often themselves placed at risk, either given into the care of families of origin in which their mothers were abused, or into a foster system which only partially protects children from abuse, and sometimes exposes them directly to it. Given that poverty and a lack of social support have been linked to greater risks of sexual abuse and criminality, the deficit in psychological services offered to women offenders risk perpetuating a familial cycle of incarceration (Marcus-Mendoza & Wright, 2004).

According to Braithwaite (1989) and Fox (1982), women released after serving their sentences are often met with public disdain, deemed social outcasts and excluded from the job market; criminality in women is even more stigmatized than criminality in men, as it is a greater violation of gender role norms for women. They are left to feel shamed and experience feelings of powerlessness, which has the potential to trigger a relapse of substance use (Bill, 1998; Browne & Finkelhor, 1986). Many of these women utilize prostitution and drug dealing as a means to support their families as well as to pay the costs of their own addictions (Bloom, Chesney-Lind & Owen, 1994) leading them into a trauma reenactment in which they are likely to be further traumatized (Farley, Cotton, Lynne, Zumbeck, Spiwak, Reyes, Alvarez, & Sezgin, 2003).

These risky lifestyles also often lead to a multitude of health complications, including risk of exposure to HIV and Hepatitis C, both of which are becoming endemic among incarcerated women. In a study by Salholz and Wright (1990), 35% of the 400 participants incarcerated at a Massachusetts prison were found to be HIV positive. A subsequent study indicated a 4% incidence of HIV among female inmates, compared to 2.3% among incarcerated males (Gowdy, Corrothers, Katsel, Parmley, & Schmidt, 1998). It is surmised that the high rate of HIV and AIDS among incarcerated females is a consequence of prostitution, intravenous drug use and multiple sexual partners, many of whom are also IV drug users (Kane & DiBartolo, 2002); all of these are, in turn, common behavioral consequences of childhood maltreatment and trauma. Health difficulties, however, are not limited to fatal diseases. Wilson and Leasure (1991) found that incarceration alone could exacerbate several medical issues including diabetes, asthma, ulcers and epilepsy, several of which are found at higher rates among women with a CSA history. Compounding these ailments is potential weight gain, which often occurs as a result of limited dietary options and hypertension (Kane & DiBartolo, 2002).

Study findings also have corroborated early evidence regarding high rates of mental health conditions and emotional difficulties among incarcerated women (Boney-McCoy & Finkelhor, 1998; Maeve, 1999). Teplin, Abram and McClelland (1996) found a 33.3% lifetime prevalence of Post Traumatic Stress Disorder among a sample of incarcerated females, which compares with a general population lifetime prevalence for women of 8% (DSM-IV-TR, 2000). In a subsequent study of incarcerated women Jordan, Schlengler, Fairbank and Caddell (1996) found that 30% of the women interviewed reported six or more symptoms of Post Traumatic Stress Disorder. Despite these figures, the primary therapeutic intervention utilized to treat the mental and emotional symptoms of female offenders is often pharmacological (Maeve, 1999), which neither we, nor any author whose work on treating complex trauma we have reviewed, see as the treatment of choice for a complex trauma picture. The Bureau of Justice Statistics (2000) indicated that approximately 20% of all female offenders received psychotropic medications subsequent to their admission, some evidence that a primarily psychopharmacological route does not adequately address the ways in which post-traumatic and dissociative features of these women's functioning puts them at risk for criminal behaviors and incarceration.

Given that a history of sexual and physical abuse drastically increases the likelihood a woman will abuse drugs and alcohol, it is not surprising that the rates of alcoholism and addiction are high among incarcerated females (Bureau of Justice Statistics, 2000; Covington, 2003). The Bureau of Justice Statistics (2000) estimated 50% of all incarcerated females confined in state prisons reported drinking alcohol and utilizing illicit drugs in the year prior to their offense. In addition, 40% of all female offenders admitted to being under the influence of drugs at the time of their offense, The National Institute of Justice's (1998) findings indicated 54% of women in prison used drugs the month before the commitment of their crime. Kerr's (1998) findings indicated of 80 incarcerated women surveyed, 12.5% reported high levels of alcohol use and 34.9% had similar levels of drug use. Slightly more than two-thirds of these offenders admitted to using multiple drugs.

Among women abuse survivors incarcerated for violent crime, there are striking commonalities in the nature of the offense they have committed. According to Phillips and Harm (1998), 36% of these women committed a violent act against an intimate, although the Bureau of Justice Statistics (2000) estimates this number to be around two-thirds. The National Institute of Justice (1998) reported that women offenders serving a sentence for a violent crime were twice as likely as their male counterparts to have had an intimate relationship with their victim. In crimes in which women killed their abusers, the majority report that they did so as a last resort in defense of their own lives and or the lives of their children (Prisoners with Children, 2005). Browne (1989), in her study of battered women who kill, describes what we would now likely call a complex trauma presentation for many of these women, including prominent dissociative symptoms occurring in the context of high-intensity present-day abuse which triggers symptoms from earlier childhood maltreatment experiences.

Given the unique profiles and needs of incarcerated females, it is imperative that attention be given to this neglected population. In addressing the needs and concerns of this vulnerable population it is likely that the psychological, physical, financial and social burden placed on the offenders, their families and society will be lessened. Our particular concern is with the failure of current correctional mental health programs to directly address the emotional, cognitive, behavioral and spiritual consequences of exposure to complex trauma, all of which we believe to be implicated both in these women's presence in the criminal justice system, as well as in their risk for future recidivism. Given the potential for women's incarceration to spread the risks of complex trauma to the second and succeeding generations, we see the development of trauma-specific interventions with these women as both an ethical imperative, and also as a strategy benefiting the larger society which now pays the costs, financial and human, of women's post-trauma symptoms emerging as criminal acts. In response to these concerns we decided to investigate whether and how a trauma-focused intervention for women inmates who are CSA survivors might make a difference in their trauma-related functioning.

Prior to our research there had been no studies on the development, implementation and outcome of trauma-based therapies conducted at the Washington Correction Center for Women, even though statistics gathered at two disparate points in time (Jordan v. Gardner; Walker, 2005; Washington Dept. of Corrections, 2005) documented that at least 65% and perhaps as high as 85% of the women entering this facility had histories of severe and repeated childhood and/or adult trauma, consistent with the national picture of incarcerated women. In fact, the first two authors, who were the experimenters on this study under the supervision of the third author, found it difficult to unearth any writing or research on this topic at all in any correctional setting dealing with women offenders in the years prior to 2005 when we first reviewed the literature. Various psychoeducational group interventions have been employed with incarcerated women; however, they have not specifically focused on childhood sexual abuse survivors. Although group treatment modalities addressing Attention Deficit Disorder, depression, interpersonal relationships and sex offenders have been developed at WCCW there has been a lack of attention given to those who have endured childhood trauma, specifically childhood sexual abuse (John Haroian, PhD, personal communication, June 2005). As a result, data regarding the effectiveness of psychotherapeutic group interventions for the treatment of female childhood sexual abuse survivors among incarcerated females were unavailable.

Due to the relevance of these issues (e.g., increased numbers of incarcerated women and budgetary constraints) we believed it important to empirically establish the effectiveness of time-limited, trauma-focused groups for incarcerated women. Our hope was that by demonstrating the effectiveness of a time-limited yet trauma-focused treatment that we would simultaneously respond to the realities of the WCCW system where resources are in short supply, as well as the needs among the women offenders. The first two authors had each worked as predoctoral practicum students at WCCW and had become very familiar with the depth of the need to offer trauma-focused treatment to the many CSA survivors incarcerated in the institution. The third author, having served as an expert witness on behalf of the WCCW inmates who sued the state of Washington in the Jordan v. Gardner case, was aware of the extent to which this population was affected by the precursors of complex trauma. Thus, like much other feminist research, this study had agendas that fit the needs of the institutional corrections system because of an implicit strategy of influencing that system via our findings. More importantly, we sought to find ways to empower trauma survivors whose experiences of complex trauma and dissociation had led to serious consequences in terms of loss of freedom, which is the ultimate form of post-traumatic disempowerment.

DESCRIPTION OF STUDY

We examined the impact of a time-limited repeated-measures group treatment intervention on female offenders' reports of distress occurring from childhood sexual abuse. Due to constraints of time and participant availability this study was preliminary in nature with a sample size not large enough to draw strongly generalizable conclusions. We adopted, instead, a goal of yielding sufficient information to serve as heuristics for future research. We developed and implemented a 16-session trauma-focused group intervention with recently incarcerated women who volunteered to participate.[1] We specifically hypothesized that this brief group intervention would reduce trauma-related symptomatology when compared to a wait-list control group. Two trauma-specific and one general measure were administered pre and post treatment. A randomly selected wait-list control group was given the same measures, and then also offered the treatments after the initial treatment group went through post-tests.

Thirteen participants were selected from a larger sample of incarcerated women at the Washington Correction Center for Women. All potential participants were initially screened upon arrival at the institution, using a brief screening questionnaire, and were subsequently screened further in an interview with the researchers. Participants in the study were included if they: (1) had a history of childhood sexual abuse, (2) were not engaged in current psychotherapy, (3) had no known or reported history of sexual deviancy, and (4) had been sentenced to a minimum of one year (so as to be available for treatment and follow-up). Offenders who met the required criteria were provided information about the study and a written informed consent was obtained from those who elected to voluntarily participate.

Because of the feminist orientation of the researchers, creating as much voluntariness as possible was important in participant selection. It is likely that we could have secured more, and more consistent, participation had we brought authority of the prison system to bear on the women. We (Cole and Sarlund-Heinrich) made a decision very early on, based on our previous work as feminist therapists practicing at WCCW, not to use any coercive means either to obtain or to keep participants. This had the problematic (for us) outcome of keeping our numbers low and our drop-out rates higher than we would have liked. However, what we have represents results from women who had the choice to be present at their treatment; thus the experimental treatment would not itself lead to a form of traumatic reenactment of disempowerment.

Participants ranged from 19 to 46 years of age with a mean age of 31 years (SD = 9.8). Thirty-three percent of participants identified as Caucasian. The remainder of the participants identified as Mexican, Native American/Caucasian, Native American, African American/Native American, Hispanic/Native American/Mexican and Hispanic/African American, with each group representing eleven percent of the total. The average years of education were 12.5. Sexual orientation characteristics were as follows: Heterosexual (77.8%), Lesbian (11.1%) and Bisexual (11.1%). With regard to marital status, 55.6% reported being single, 11.1% married, 22.2% divorced and 11.1% widowed.

Measures

All participants completed four instruments and a demographic questionnaire. Since one instrument (the Brief Symptom Inventory-BSI) is a short form of another (the SCL-90-R) we will combine the data on those two instruments, which were both included for research purposes as tests of general psychological functioning. The Symptom Checklist-90-Revised (SCL-90-R) is a 90-item self-report symptom inventory of current, point-in-time, psychological symptom status, designed to reflect the psychological symptom patterns of community, medical, and psychiatric respondents (Derogatis, 1994). Raw scores for the nine dimensions and three global indices are converted into standard T scores based on a distribution with a mean of 50 and a standard deviation of 10. As a whole, the SCL-90-R is a good test to assess for current psychological symptomatology (different than the TSI which assesses for psychological symptomatology over the last six months), particularly as it has been found to adequately detect symptoms of distress in patients with and without histories of abuse (Bryer, Nelson, Miller, & Krol, 1987; Swett, Surrey, & Cohen, 1999). Test-retest reliability of the SCL-90-R across two studies suggests coefficients ranging from .66 (for Somatization) to .90 after a ten-week and a two-week lapse between test intervals, respectively (Derogatis, Rickels, & Rock, 1976; Horowitz, Rosenberg, Baer, Ureno, & Villasenor, 1988).

We also administered the Trauma Symptom Inventory (TSI), a 100-item questionnaire which assesses possible post-trauma symptoms. The TSI has the ability to assess for a wide range of psychological effects in addition to intra- and interpersonal difficulties often associated with trauma sequelae (Briere, 1995). Respondents' individual responses are transformed from raw scale scores into T scores with a mean of 50 and a standard deviation of 10. T scores at or above 65 are considered clinically significant. TSI scales are internally consistent at .86, .87, .84, and .84 in a general population, a clinical population, a university population, and a military population, respectively (Briere, 1995). Additionally, the TSI has demonstrated convergent, predictive, and incremental validity in a number of studies (Briere & Elliott, 1998; Runtz & Roche, 1999; Shapiro & Schwartz, 1997).

Finally, utilizing a projective measure, we administered the Rorschach Inkblot Method (RIM). The RIM consists of ten bilaterally symmetrical inkblots. Subjects are asked to articulate their perception of the inkblot when presented to them by the examiner. Each individual perception identified by the subject is considered a unique and separate response. The sum of these responses makes up the overall total number of responses, which are used as both a validity measure and calculation for various components of the RIM. Once the responses have been recorded they are scored according to three general categories: (1) location; (2) determinants; and (3) content (Groth-Marnat, 1997). Various norms have been established for the RIM, however the ones utilized in this study can be found in Exner (2003) and are currently the most widely accepted norms for scoring and interpretation of this instrument. For the purpose of this study the Trauma Content Index (TC/R) (Armstrong &

Lowenstein, 1990) was utilized as a second trauma-specific measure. The TC/R is the sum of five of the twenty-seven total content scores of the RIM (blood, anatomy, sex, aggression and morbid) divided by the total number of responses.

Procedure

Participants were randomly assigned to treatment or no-treatment comparison groups by drawing numbers from a box. For the treatment group, the TSI, the SCL-90-R and the Rorschach were completed prior to the first session and immediately following the conclusion of treatment. The control group took all tests at the same time as the women in the treatment group. The treatment group initially consisted of seven members; however, one dropped out before testing began and two additional members dropped out of the treatment group in session two. The final number of group members in the treatment group was four. The control group consisted of six members, with one leaving prior to the post-test.

The treatment group met bi-weekly for 2.5 hours for a total of 8 weeks. Based on our review of interventions likely to be helpful to women CSA survivors (Brown, Schefflin, & Hammond, 1998; Harris 1998; Herman, 1992; Lewis, Kelly & Allen, 2004), a four phase treatment approach was employed. The four phases included: (1) self-soothing and safety, (2) psychoeducation, (3) processing, and (4) termination. The first seven sessions focused on boundary setting, self-esteem and identity, and relaxation (Briere, 1992; Lewis, Kelly & Allen). Sessions eight through eleven focused on understanding trauma and sexual abuse, trauma and addiction, identifying interpersonal patterns of abuse and assertiveness training (Harris, 1998). Session twelve focused on the processing and writing of personal stories of trauma. Members engaged in a full hour of writing their personal story of childhood sexual abuse.

Immediately following the writing exercise, participants were given the opportunity to openly discuss the writing experience. Before ending the session, relaxation and self-soothing strategies were employed. In addition, participants shredded the personal stories written to ensure confidentiality (as any materials taken back to a cell were subject to search and seizure by prison staff at any time, for no reason). The last four sessions consisted of processing and termination. The group was facilitated by the first author. Treatment adherence was assessed using therapist's case notes and journaling following each session.

Participants who were assigned to the wait-list control group were informed of their option to receive group treatment upon the completion of the study. All participants in this group elected to participate in treatment, with one leaving prior to the fourth session.

RESULTS

Demographic information and TSI, SCL-90-R, and Rorschach scores are found in Tables 1 and 2. First, the scores indicate the presence of both post traumatic symptomatology as well as dissociative symptoms among both the treatment and control groups, throughout the sixteen weeks covered by the study. Mean scores for the treatment group (44.25 to 63.7) as well as the control group (62.2 to 75) on the ten clinical scales of the TSI are indicative of trauma symptomatology. Consistent with these results are the TCI mean scores of the Rorschach. At pre-test, the treatment group yielded a mean score of .28 and the control group a mean score of .26, which indicates the presence of trauma symptomatology in both groups.

Decreases were found in the mean Trauma Content (TC/R) scores of the Rorschach Inkblot Method (RIM) from the pre- to the post-treatment measure. There were no apparent changes from pre- to post-treatment on the TSI and the SCL-90-R. In addition, comparisons between the treatment and the control group also suggest no differences, with the possible exception of the Somatization and the Phobic Anxiety scales of the SCL-90-R. Inspection of the data from the wait-list control group showed a decline in scores, all in the direction of greater severity and more symptoms during the period of time in which the treatment group's scores remained the same. Thus, although our initial research hypotheses were that treatment would lead to change, what we found, instead, is that it is likely that treatment at this point in incarceration (e.g., immediately at intake) prevented an aggravation of symptoms that is more typical among newly incarcerated women with a history of CSA.

On the last day of the treatment group, participants were allowed to evaluate the material used and the therapist. Group members overwhelmingly reported that they believed the group was beneficial and they reported that they would go away with more effective coping skills. In particular, they felt that the handouts were helpful; for instance, a handout with the definitions of all the terms we were using assisted the women with gaining a better understanding of trauma. They asked for

TABLE 1. Demographic Information

Scale/Condition	Control		Treatment	
	Frequency	Percent	Frequency	Percent
Current age				
19 Years of Age	0	0	1	25
22 Years of Age	0	0	1	25
27 Years of Age	2	40	2	50
39 Years of Age	1	20	0	0
45 Years of Age	1	20	0	0
46 Years of Age	1	20	0	0
Ethnicity				
Caucasian	2	40	1	25
Mexican	1	20	0	0
Native American/Caucasian	1	20	0	0
Native American	1	20	0	0
African American/ Native American	0	0	1	25
Hispanic/Native American/Mexican	0	0	1	25
Hispanic/African American	0	0	1	25
Sexual orientation				
Heterosexual	4	80	3	75
Lesbian	1	20	0	0
Bisexual	0	0	1	20
Marital status				
Single	2	40	3	75
Married	0	0	1	25
Divorced	2	40	0	0
Widow	1	20	0	0
Years of education				
11 Years or less	0	0	1	25
12 Years	2	40	2	50
13 Years of More	3	60	1	25
Reason for incarceration				
Forgery	1	20	0	0
First Degree Assault	0	0	1	25
Possession/Escape/ Bail Jumping/Burglary Attempted Robbery	3	60	1	25
Second Degree Theft or Burglary	0	0	0	0

Scale/Condition	Control		Treatment	
	Frequency	Percent	Frequency	Percent
Violated Restraining Order	0	0	1	25
Promoting Prostitution	1	20	0	0
Number of times incarcerated				
1 Time	2	40	3	75
2 Times	1	20	1	25
3 Times	1	20	0	0
4 or More Times	1	20	0	0
Length of incarceration				
1-12 Months	1	20	0	0
13-45 Months	2	40	1	50
46-84 Months	2	40	0	0
85-168 Months	0	0	2	50
Age sexually abused				
0-2 Years of Age	2	40	1	25
3-5 Years of Age	1	20	2	50
6-12 Years of Age	2	60	1	25
Who touched you sexually				
Male Family Member	3	60	2	50
Family Friend	1	20	0	0
Mother's Boyfriend	0	0	1	25
Babysitter	1	20	1	25
Were you sexually abused by more than one individual in childhood?				
Yes	3	60	4	100
No	2	40	0	0
How many people sexually abused you?				
1 Time	2	40	0	0
2-3 Times	2	40	3	75
5 or More Times	1	20	1	25
Ever sexually abused as an adult?				
Yes	2	40	1	25
No	3	60	3	75
Ever received therapy as a child or adult?				
Yes	4	80	2	50
No	1	20	2	50
Ever received group therapy in prison or out of prison?				
Yes	2	40	2	50
No	3	60	2	50
Are you currently taking mental helth medications?				
Yes	5	100	1	25
No	0	0	3	75

Note: N = 5 for Control Group; N = 4 for Treatment Group.

TABLE 2. Pre and Post Mean Scores on Dependent Measures

| Scale/Condition | Control | | | | Treatment | | | |
| | Pretest | | Posttest | | Pretest | | Posttest | |
	Mean	(SD)	Mean	(SD)	Mean	(SD)	Mean	(SD)
Trauma Content Index	.27	(.33)	.28	(.33)	.29	(.21)	.07	(.05)
Trauma Symptom Inventory								
Atypical Response	72.8	(19.6)	70.8	(22.8)	60.3	(7.4)	55.5	(9.6)
Response Level	42.0	(2.2)	42.0	(2.2)	52.0	(9.9)	49.5	(7.0)
Inconsistent Response	50.0	(3.0)	53.0	(10.7)	51.5	(10.5)	47.5	(7.7)
Anxious Arousal	67.2	(8.1)	70.6	(6.9)	54.5	(13.2)	50.0	(3.5)
Depression	62.6	(13.6)	66.2	(9.7)	58.0	(13.0)	55.75	(12.2)
Anger/Irritibility	57.2	(8.6)	66.6	(4.6)	44.4	(8.8)	44.5	(5.1)
Intrusive Experiences	73.6	(11.5)	75.4	(7.1)	63.8	(16.4)	62.3	(10.5)
Defensive Avoidance	70.0	(7.3)	72.2	(4.9)	60.0	(10.1)	59.5	(8.0)
Dissociation	74.6	(12.3)	74.6	(16.0)	63.5	(14.3)	55.5	(10.4)
Sexual Concerns	65.2	(12.1)	70.6	(16.1)	44.5	(2.5)	43.5	(3.0)
Dysfunctional Sexual Behavior	75.0	(23.2)	83.8	(18.5)	44.8	(1.5)	44.0	(0.0)
Impaired Self Reference	64.6	(12.8)	70.0	(9.6)	51.8	(8.9)	49.0	(6.8)
Tension Reduction Behavior	67.2	(18.9)	78.8	(22.0)	44.3	(2.9)	44.3	(2.9)
Symptom Checklist-90-R								
Somatization	66.0	(7.2)	77.0	(7.9)	52.8	(2.8)	54.5	(7.9)
Obsessive-Compulsive	60.6	(7.1)	77.0	(3.8)	51.5	(14.3)	61.5	(13.3)
Interpersonal Sensitivity	53.0	(11.3)	70.6	(15.3)	45.0	(11.9)	58.3	(6.7)
Depression	56.4	(13.0)	76.0	(6.9)	46.3	(8.3)	61.0	(15.0)
Anxiety	58.4	(7.6)	77.4	(4.9)	44.8	(8.8)	59.8	(9.2)
Hostility	49.8	(7.3)	67.0	(7.1)	41.3	(8.3)	47.5	(5.8)
Phobic Anxiety	56.2	(10.8)	71.8	(6.8)	46.3	(5.9)	48.8	(9.5)
Paranoid Ideation	55.6	(5.8)	74.8	(5.7)	52.8	(8.9)	61.8	(6.2)
Psychoticism	56.4	(10.4)	77.6	(6.5)	50.6	(13.3)	61.5	(12.6)
Global Severity Index	59.4	(9.9)	76.8	(5.8)	47.25	(10.4)	60.5	(8.7)
Positive Symptom Distress Index	57.6	(11.6)	75.2	(7.6)	48.0	(10.1)	61.3	(8.8)
Positive Symptom Total	60.4	(10.5)	74.4	(6.3)	47.5	(9.3)	58.3	(9.2)

Note: N = 5 for Control Group; N = 4 for Treatment Group.

extra handouts on the definitions so they could share them with their family members. The women said the group assisted them in understanding that they were not alone. Additionally, the women liked that they were considered the "expert" of their lived experience and they felt empowered to share those experiences. We had similar feedback from the members of the wait-list control group when they received the treatment intervention. It was clear from what our participants told us that their subjective perceptions of this intervention were that it made a difference for them because, often for the first time in their lives, someone had given voice and a name to their experiences and had begun the process of empowering them to make connections between their having been victimized and the problematic coping strategies that put them on the path to prison.

DISCUSSION

It is clear from the literature discussed previously that early exposure to childhood sexual abuse has many detrimental effects on a person's adult functioning. Research seems to suggest that a combination of factors plays a more important role in the development and maintenance of symptomatology than any one factor alone. This is particularly true in the case of the very large numbers of women who are incarcerated, most of whom have histories of multiple forms of trauma in their lives (e.g., CSA, rape, domestic violence, etc.). Incarcerated women are a neglected population; typically, the few treatment and/or programs provided to them are based upon programs that are available to incarcerated men, and almost always fail to take into account women's roles or their biology, all of which may affect both vulnerability to, and response to, trauma.

In the present study, we piloted an effort to rectify this long-standing neglect with a program that met bi-weekly for 2.5 hours for a total of 8 weeks. The group drew upon the literature on trauma treatment, and used primarily psychoeducational strategies for teaching healthy coping skills such as boundary setting, healthy self-soothing, self-esteem enhancement, and relaxation techniques. The group attended to normalizing women's experiences of shame and identity impairment, and assisted in the development of strategies for managing histories of past trauma in an empowering manner. Although there were few apparent changes due to treatment found in this study, results did indicate that the 16-session treatment modality utilized may have prevented the exacerbation of symptomatology among participants in the treatment group. We see this as an important finding; although typically incarceration makes women more symptomatic, our intervention was able to prevent that outcome for these women, thus decreasing the likelihood of a difficult adjustment to their prison experience. These results have been effective in establishing a foundation for future research utilizing a time-limited group modality for incarcerated women with CSA.

Anecdotal evidence from the groups treated in the current study, as well as anecdotal findings from other our extensive other contacts with women in the prison in our roles as treatment providers or evaluators, suggests that women's specific gendered roles, particularly in the context of the reenactment of traumatogenic interpersonal relationships, appear to emerge repeatedly in their personal narratives. The women who participated in this group were able to demonstrate effective coping strategies, including self-restraint and advocacy, as a result of new skills learned in the group; these women avidly embraced this new learning. For example, one member reported to us that as a result of the group, she was able to refrain from engaging in physical altercations on three separate occasions, which is quite extraordinary given her extensive prior history of assault charges. A second group member acted as an advocate when she reported the predatory and sexually abusive behavior of a fellow inmate. For this woman to speak out in this manner and see herself as having the right to be protected from sexual predation rather than seeing it as her normal life was a striking change for her. Even within the constraints of the prison environment, our group participants reported experiencing many of the same sorts of treatment benefits as those reported by clients receiving CSA-focused treatment in non-prison clinical contexts (Brown, Schefflin, & Hammond, 1998; Harris,1998; Herman, 1992; Lewis, Kelly, & Allen, 2004). For women in prison these changes seem even more important; their use of post-traumatic dissociative coping strategies has literally endangered their lives and cost them their freedom.

Given the mixed results of this study in regard to changes on the instruments used to assess outcomes, it is important to examine the potential explanations of our findings. Some of our mixed findings are likely to reflect the difference between what is measured by objective and projective instruments, which in turn may give us clues as to how to better understand the change process for CSA survivors. The Trauma Symptom Inventory (TSI) and the Symptom Checklist-90-Revised (SCL-90-R) are somewhat face valid instruments which may affect outcome scores at pre-test and post-test. Additionally, these instruments both measure the presence of overt symptoms and behaviors, which may not evince immediate change in response to a short-term treatment strategy. The Rorschach Inkblot Method (RIM) in contrast, is a projective measure that assesses unconscious processes such as cognitive schemas and personality structure. Although the Rorschach Inkblot Method does not contain specific scales to assess under- or over-reporting, the ambiguity of the instrument makes it virtually impossible for participants to manipulate responses. This may indicate that trauma-related unconscious processes may have decreased, even while overall symptomatologies, including specific symptoms associated both with PTSD and complex trauma, have not. It is our sense that this theory best explains our findings; the changes occurring as a result of our brief treatment intervention are more subtle, and thus more likely to be detected by an instrument that focuses away from specific symptoms. This notion is consistent with psychodynamic theory, the foundation of projective assessment, which holds fast to the idea that information learned first affects unconscious processes and then conscious processes. Given this rationale, if the therapeutic information gleaned by participants was to have initially impacted primarily or only unconscious processes, changes would not have been accurately assessed by the TSI and the SCL-90-R, which measures conscious overt symptoms, at the time of post-test.

An additional explanation for the differences found may be related to time constraints and lack of a secondary post-test follow-up. Given that the only post-test measure occurred immediately following the conclusion of the group, participants may have not been provided adequate time to utilize and integrate effective coping skills and thus to experience changes in behaviors and expressed symptoms. Thus an overall measure of specific symptomatology, such as the TSI and SCL-90-R may have not demonstrated a decrease.

As noted above findings from the SCL-90-R and the TSI indicated that the treatment group scores did not change from pre-test to post-test, indicating that trauma symptoms remained constant and did not exacerbate. In contrast the scores of the wait list control group worsened over the same time period. These results may signify that although 16 sessions of treatment did not lead to a decrease in symptomatology, the treatment did prevent symptoms from intensifying. Aggravation of symptoms and increase in problematic behaviors appears to be the norm for women on the intake unit at WCCW, according to our and other staff members' observations; our data confirm these impressions. It is distinctly possible that what looks like no change in a non-incarcerated sample–e.g., no decrease of symptoms–may represent a good outcome in an incarcerated sample–e.g., the prevention of a normative increase of symptoms. Findings from our assessment of the women in the wait list control group indicated that post traumatic symptomatology as well as dissociative symptoms had a tendency to intensify during the eight weeks of no treatment. If as a result of a trauma-focused treatment women entering prison do not increase in their post-traumatic and dissociative coping strategies, but rather remain constant, even with such brief treatment, then the potential benefit from longer-term treatment, or treatment offered repeatedly during the course of incarceration rather than only at intake, is great. If nothing else, achieving these outcomes from an initial intervention may instill hope in these women that change is possible, and that post-traumatic growth may result from therapeutic work during incarceration.

Our sense is that in order to accurately assess the effectiveness of such an intervention we might need to design measures that are specific to the manner in which trauma is reenacted by women who are incarcerated. Longer-term follow-up of our clients to determine how and whether they were able to utilize and deepen their new coping strategies during the course of their incarceration would also be an important direction to take for further research with this group.

Study Limitations

As with all preliminary investigations it is important to acknowledge the limitations of this investigation. There were a number of limitations to this preliminary investigation which included: (1) small sample size, (2) use of volunteer participants and consequent effects on generalizability, (3) extraneous variables, (4) post-treatment assessment, and (5) limited resources available to the researchers.

A primary limitation of this study was the small sample size. Due to institutional constraints, which slowed the process of IRB approval and time frames constraining the work of the researchers, the recruiting of participants for this study was time limited. These constraints, coupled with offender scheduling conflicts, prevented us from obtaining a larger sample size. A second limitation of this study was the inclusion of only volunteer participants housed in the receiving unit of the prison. Results from this preliminary investigation can only be generalized to similar groups of women at WCCW.

Another limitation of the study can be attributed to multiple environmental variables. This study did not control for age, drug and alcohol histories, other forms of abuse, length of incarceration, medication regimen, or comorbid disorders. The disparity of these variables may explain the variation in test score data.

A fourth limitation is the lack of post-test follow-up at a specified secondary interval. Due to time constraints, a second post-test follow-up could not occur. The inability to perform a secondary follow-up may have directly impacted outcome data. Adding a secondary post-test follow-up could have potentially improved outcome scores by providing participants with more time to utilize skills acquired and time to integrate these skills into their coping repertoire.

Finally, the first two authors, who conducted this research, were constrained due to limitations on their resources. As doctoral students conducting dissertation research in the context of no funding support, our ability to extend our work beyond its initial stages was limited.

CONCLUSIONS

Women traumatized repeatedly as children, a characteristic common to the histories of incarcerated women, often cope with their post-traumatic symptoms via trauma reenactments, many of which place them at risk for being convicted of a crime. Almost every woman who came into WCCW during our time working there had been in multiple abusive intimate relationships as an adult, and often their most recent relationship was the precipitant for the crimes for which they were convicted and incarcerated. Data and anecdotal evidence emerging from this experience would argue for more gender-specific research on women in prison and their experience of trauma, as well as gender-aware strategies for treatment, consistent with the recommendations of APA's Guidelines for Psychotherapy with Girls and Women (Nutt, Rice, & Enns, 2002).

Given the lack of empirical research substantiating effective group treatment for incarcerated females with a history of CSA, we believe that additional research regarding effective trauma-focused therapies with this population is needed.

Even from this limited sample, it is clear to us that an effective trauma-focused treatment intervention is needed for incarcerated women. Post-traumatic dissociative coping strategies, particularly the use of drugs as a means of numbing and distancing from painful affects, are among the most powerful factors placing a number of these women on the path to prison, and these coping strategies re-assert themselves when these women leave prison untreated. The findings of this investigation emphasize the real possibility for therapeutic change among incarcerated female survivors of CSA. Even a brief intervention such as ours made a difference for some of our participants and created the expectation that change was possible, and that other coping strategies for managing painful affects might be available. It is also becoming more clear from these findings that neglect of CSA survivors' trauma-specific problems will not be a case of "doing no harm" by doing nothing. Rather, our data suggest that for this population, post-traumatic and dissociative symptoms increase as women are exposed to the highly stressful environment of a prison intake unit, a setting in which the locus of control is sharply shifted out of their hands. To avoid aggravating the post-traumatic symptoms with which this population enters the corrections system, an active, trauma-focused intervention is necessary.

For change to occur in systems that incarcerate women offenders it is imperative that a therapeutic model similar to the one utilized in this study be employed as a strategy for reducing the on-going effects of childhood trauma. Without proper allocations of funds, adequate training and a commitment from prison administrators who control what occurs in their institutions, the negative repercussions of CSA will continue in these women's lives; their symptoms will aggravate, leading to more difficulties for them during the course of their incarceration as well as vulnerability to re-offending once released. This perpetuating cycle will have ongoing consequences for not only the women incarcerated but for society as a whole. A call to action is needed on a community, state and national level if we are to make a difference in the lives of incarcerated female survivors of CSA.

NOTE

1. A copy of the manual for this intervention is available from the first authors.

REFERENCES

Acklin, M. W., McDowell, C. J., Verschell, M. S., & Chan, D. (2002). Interobservor agreement, intraobservor reliability, and the Rorschach Comprehensive System. *Journal of Personality Assessment, 74*, 15-47.

American Psychiatric Association. (1994). *Diagnostic and statistical manual of mental disorders* (4th ed.). Washington, DC: Author.

Armstrong, J. G., & Lowenstein, R. J. (1990). Characteristics of patient with multiple personality and dissociative disorders on psychological testing. *Journal of Nervous and Mental Disorders, 178*, 448-454.

Bill, L. (1998). The victimization and revictimization of female offenders: Prison administrators should be aware of way in which security procedures perpetrate feelings of powerlessness among incarcerated women. *Corrections Today, 60*(7), 106-108.

Bloom, S. (1997). *Creating sanctuary: Toward an evolution of sane societies.* New York: Guilford Press.

Bloom, B., Chesney-Lind, M., & Owen, B. (1994). *Women in California prisons: Hidden victims of the war on drugs.* San Francisco: Center on Juvenile and Criminal Justice.

Boney-McCoy, S., & Finkelhor, D. (1998). Psychopathology associated with sexual abuse: A reply to Nash, Neimeyer, Hulsey and Lambert. [Electronic version]. *Journal of Consulting and Clinical Psychology, 66*(3), 1-4.

Bradley, R. G., & Davino, K. M. (2002). Women's perceptions of the prison environment: When prison is "the safest place I've ever been." [Electronic version]. *Psychology of Women Quarterly, 26*, 351-359.

Braithwaite, J. (1989). *Crime, shame and reintegration.* Cambridge, UK: Cambridge University Press.

Briere, J. (1992). *Clinical abuse trauma: Theory and treatment of the lasting effects.* Newbury Park, CA: Sage.

Briere, J. (1995). *Traumatic Symptom Inventory: Professional manual.* Florida: Psychological Assessment Resources, Inc.

Brown, D., Schefflin, A. W., & Hammond, D. C. (1998). *Memory, trauma, treatment and the law.* New York: W.W. Norton.

Browne, A. (1989). *When battered women kill.* New York, NY: Free Press.

Browne, A., & Finkelhor, D. (1986). Impact of sexual abuse: A review of the research. *Psychological Bulletin, 99*, 66-77.

Browne, A., Miller, B., & Maguin, E. (1999). Prevalence and severity of lifetime physical and sexual victimization among incarcerated women. [Electronic version]. *International Journal of Law and Psychiatry, 22*, 301-322.

Bureau of Justice Statistics. (2000). *Women offenders, 1999*, NCJ-175688. Washington, DC: U.S. Department of Justice.

Bureau of Justice Statistics (2002). *Incarcerated women in the United States: Facts and figures.* Washington, DC: U.S. Department of Justice.

Bureau of Justice Statistics (2005). *Prison statistics.* Washington, DC: U.S. Department of Justice.

Cerney, M. (1990). The Rorschach and traumatic loss: Can the presence of traumatic loss be detected from the Rorschach? *Journal of Personality Assessment, 55*, 781-789.

Courtois, C. A. (1997). Healing the incest wound: A treatment update with attention to recovered-memory issues. [Electronic Version]. *American Journal of Psychotherapy, 51*, 464-497.

Courtois, C. (2004). Complex trauma, complex reactions: Assessment and treatment. [Electronic Version]. *Psychotherapy: Theory, Research, Practice, Training, 41*, 412-425.

Covington, S. S. (1998). Women in prison: Approaches in treatment of our most invisible population. [Electronic version]. *Women and Therapy Journal, 21*, 141-155.

Covington, S. S. (2003). *A women's journey home: Challenges for female offenders.* Retrieved January 21, 2005 from http://www.stephaniecovington.com/html/journey.html.

Derogatis, L. R. (1994). *SCL-90-R Symptom Checklist-90-R: Administration, scoring, and procedures manual* (3rd ed.). Minnesota: NCS Pearson, Inc.

Dodge, M., & Pogrebin, M. R. (2001). Collateral costs of imprisonment for women: Complications of reintegration. [Electronic version]. *The Prison Journal, 81,* 42-54.

Elmone, P., & Lingg, M. A. (1996). Adult survivors of sexual trauma: A conceptualization for treatment. [Electronic Version]. *Journal of Mental Health Counseling, 18,* 108-123.

Exner, J. E., Jr. (2003). *The Rorschach: A comprehensive system* (4th ed.). New Jersey: Wiley & Sons, Inc.

Fox, J. (1982). Women in prison: A case study in the social reality of *stress.* In R. Johnson & H. Toch (Eds.), *The pains of imprisonment* (pp. 205-220). Beverly Hills, CA: Sage.

Gowdy, V. B., Cain, T., Corrothers, H., Katsel, T. H., Parmley, A. M., & Schmidt, A. (1998). *Women in the justice system–A twenty year update.* Washington, DC: National Institute of Justice.

Harris, M. (1998). *Trauma recovery and empowerment: A clinician's guide for working with women in groups.* New York: The Free Press.

Herman, J. L. (1992). *Trauma and recovery: The aftermath of violence–From domestic violence to political terror* (2nd ed.). New York: Basic Books.

Hunsley, J., & Bailey, J. M. (2001). Whither the Rorschach? An analysis of the evidence. *Psychological Assessment, 13,* 472-485.

Jordan, B. K., Schlenger, W. E., Fairbank, J. A., & Cadell, J. M. (1996). Prevalence of psychiatric disorders among incarcerated women: II. Convicted felons entering prisons. *Archives of General Psychiatry, 53,* 513-519.

Kane, M., & DiBartolo, M. (2002). Complex physical and mental health needs of rural incarcerated women. [Electronic version]. *Issues in Mental Health Nursing, 23,* 209-229.

Kerr, D. (1998). Substance abuse among female offenders. [Electronic version]. *Corrections Today, 60,* 114-119.

Levin, P. (1993). Assessing post traumatic stress disorder with the Rorschach projective technique. In J. P. Wilson & B. Raphaeil (Eds.), *International handbook of traumatic stress syndrome* (pp. 189-200). New York: Plenum.

Lewis, L., Kelly, K., & Allen, J. G. (2004). *Restoring hope and trust: An illustrated guide to mastering trauma.* Baltimore: The Sidran Institute Press.

Maeve, M. K. (1999). Adjudicated health: Incarcerated women and the social construction of health. *Law, Crime & Social Change, 31*(1), 49-71.

Maeve, M. K. (2000). Speaking unavoidable truths: Understanding early childhood sexual and physical violence among women in prison. [Electronic version]. *Issues in Mental Health Nursing, 21,* 473-498.

Marcus-Mendoza, S., & Wright, E. (2004). Decontextualizing female criminality: Treating abused women in prison in the United States. *Feminism and Psychology, 14,* 250-255.

Meyer, G. J., & Archer, R. P. (2001). The hard science of Rorschach research: What do we know and where do we go? *Psychological Assessment, 13,* 486-502.

National Institute of Justice (1998). *Women offenders: Programming needs and promising approaches,* 1998, NCJ-171668. Washington, DC: U.S. Department of Justice.

Nutt, R., Rice, J. K., & Enns, C. Z. (2002). *Guidelines for psychological practice with girls and women.* Washington, DC: American Psychological.

Phillips, S. D., & Harm, N. J. (1997). Women prisoners: A contextual framework. *Women and Therapy, 20,* 1-9.

Prisoners with Children (2005). *Women prisoners: Facts and figures at a glance.* Retrieved March 8, 2005 from http://www.prisoneerswithchildren.org.

Robinson, T. L. (2000). Making the hurt go away: Psychological and spiritual healing for African American women survivors of childhood incest. [Electronic Version]. *Journal of Multicultural Counseling & Development, 28,.*160-177.

Salholz, E., & Wright, L. (1990). Women in jail: Unequal Justice. [Electronic Version]. *Newsweek 51,* 37-38.

State of Washington Department of Corrections (2001). *Cost of corrections.* Retrieved February 2, 2005 from http://www.wa.gov/doc/content/faq/cost_correct.htm.

State of Washington Department of Corrections (2005). *Corrections statistics.* Retrieved August 10, 2005, from http://www.wa.gov/doc/content/secstat.htm.

Teplin, L. A., Abran, K. M., & McClelland, G. M. (1996). Prevalence of psychiatric disorders among incarcerated women: I. Pretrial detainees. *Archives of General Psychiatry, 53*(6), 505-512.

Wallis, D. A. N. (2002). Reduction of symptoms following group therapy. [Electronic version]. *Australian and New Zealand Journal of Psychiatry, 36,* 67-74.

Walker, R. (2005, August). *Intake statistics.* Paper presented at the meeting of the Washington Corrections Center for Women Mental Health Department, Gig Harbor, WA.

Wilson, J. S., & Leasure, R. (1991). Cruel and unusual punishment: The health care of women in prison. [Electronic Version]. *Nurse Practioner, 16,* 33-39.

Women's Prison Association (2003). *The population of women in prison increases rapidly.* Retrieved August 10, 2005, from http://www.wpaonline.org/resources/publications.htm.

Wood, J. M., Nezwoski, M. T., & Stejaskal, W. J. (1996). The comprehensive system for the Rorschach: A critical examination. *Psychological Science, 7,* 3-10.

doi:10.1300/J229v08n02_07

Through the Bullet-Proof Glass: Conducting Research in Prison Settings

Kathryn Quina, PhD
Ann Varna Garis, PhD
John Stevenson, PhD
Maria Garrido, PsyD
Jody Brown, PhD
Roberta Richman, MFA
Jeffrey Renzi, MS
Judith Fox, JD
Kimberly Mitchell, PhD

SUMMARY. A team of academic researchers, clinicians, prison administrators and undergraduate and graduate students came together to conduct an evaluation of a pre-release discharge planning program in a women's prison facility. This paper describes differences between academic and corrections systems, adaptations needed in order to work within the correctional system, pragmatic and ethical issues addressed by our team, and the joys and benefits we experienced doing the project. Team members who had not previously worked in a prison setting found

Kathryn Quina, Ann Varna Garis, John Stevenson, Maria Garrido, and Jody Brown are affiliated with the Department of Psychology, University of Rhode Island.

Roberta Richman, Jeffrey Renzi, and Judith Fox are affiliated with Rhode Island Department of Corrections.

Kimberly Mitchell is affiliated with Crimes Against Children Research Center, University of New Hampshire.

[Haworth co-indexing entry note]: "Through the Bullet-Proof Glass: Conducting Research in Prison Settings." Quina, Kathryn et al. Co-published simultaneously in *Journal of Trauma & Dissociation* (The Haworth Medical Press, an imprint of The Haworth Press, Inc.) Vol. 8, No. 2, 2007, pp. 123-139; and: *Trauma and Dissociation in Convicted Offenders: Gender, Science, and Treatment Issues* (ed: Kathryn Quina, and Laura S. Brown) The Haworth Medical Press, an imprint of The Haworth Press, Inc., 2007, pp. 123-139. Single or multiple copies of this article are available for a fee from The Haworth Document Delivery Service [1-800-HAWORTH, 9:00 a.m. - 5:00 p.m. (EST). E-mail address: docdelivery@haworthpress.com].

Available online at http://jtd.haworthpress.com
doi:10.1300/J229v08n02_08

it an extraordinary, transformative learning experience in spite of the challenges. doi:10.1300/J229v08n02_08 *[Article copies available for a fee from The Haworth Document Delivery Service: 1-800- HAWORTH. E-mail address: <docdelivery@haworthpress.com> Website: <http://www. HaworthPress.com>* © 2007 by The Haworth Press, Inc. All rights reserved.]

KEYWORDS. Prison system, program evaluation, ethics

INTRODUCTION

About a decade ago a group of university-based researchers and clinicians, undergraduate and graduate students, and prison administrators and staff came together for a remarkable experience. The story we offer here is not a clinical report, nor a presentation of data. Rather, we offer our experiences journeying beyond the razor wires and "through the bullet-proof glass," in hopes of informing potential researchers and clinicians about the kinds of issues they may confront, identifying important ethical and pragmatic considerations for those hoping to work within prison systems, and encouraging others to take the same journey.

BACKGROUND

The setting for this journey is the smallest state, Rhode Island, where towns and counties send anyone staying overnight in custody to one Department of Corrections campus consisting of men's and women's facilities of varying levels of security, including those awaiting trial as well as sentenced offenders. This provides a convenient arrangement for those wishing to study corrections, since a wide variety of participants are available in one place. Located close to some of the most prestigious health-related research programs in the U.S., the setting has also been ideal for intervention research in several health areas, notably addressing substance abuse, HIV risk, and PTSD, as is evident from two other papers in this volume.

In 1988, only 87 women were incarcerated in Rhode Island; two decades later, largely thanks to the "War on Drugs" which incarcerates more users for longer periods of time, 200-250 women are housed in one of two buildings (minimum and medium security) at any time. Their crimes range from prostitution and drug use to murder, but of the

148 offenders already sentenced at the time we began our work, the vast majority (70%) were repeat offenders sentenced to serve fewer than 6 months, for offenses classified as nonviolent (e.g., prostitution, using or selling drugs, or such actions as writing bad checks to purchase drugs). In reality, whatever their controlling offense, most of the women told us they had engaged in both drug use and sex work. Only 34 women (23%) were sentenced for offenses classified as violent, and many of their offenses involved substance use.

The Director of the Women's Facility, Warden Roberta Richman, had long studied and practiced feminist ethics and social justice alongside criminology and criminal justice. She sought to enable inmates to use their time productively in programs that could teach them skills, help them understand their problem behaviors, and recover from alcohol and drug addictions. Engaging the community in this process, the staff had established a "discharge planning program" which included a variety of opportunities for women to learn how to make positive changes in their lives (Box 1). A steady stream of volunteer and paid staff came to the prison to deliver these programs, which drew heavily from community agencies that could provide continuing services for women after they were released.

We formed a collaborative partnership to pursue an evaluation study of the discharge planning process. However, our personal and professional goals reflected very different perspectives. Prison officials sought feedback to inform their decision-making about resource utilization in an ever-underfunded enterprise, refining existing programs and procedures as well as identifying unmet needs. University-based researchers, in a somewhat entrepreneurial way, sought to develop and conduct an effective evaluation in such a way that students would be well trained for future careers, and researchers would have access to information that could be analyzed for publication. The clash of values inherent in bringing together two such large systems is shown in Table 1. Individuals on the team had even more disparate goals; for example, evidence that the programs helped reduce recidivism would help the Director garner administrative and staff support for her programming. One of the researchers (KQ) was interested in a specific research topic, the relationship between childhood trauma and adult HIV risk, and inmates were known to be at high risk for both. Our clinicians (AVG and MG) hoped to put together practica with incarcerated clients for doctoral students in a clinical psychology training program.

Evaluation research cannot be done in a vacuum. Researchers must establish trusting, collaborative relationships with stakeholders at

BOX 1. Discharge Planning at the RIDOC Women's Facility[1]

The discharge planning process was based on the corrections literature and informed by a feminist perspective. Assumptions behind the programming included:

- *Time spent in prison should be viewed as a window of opportunity for women to make changes in their lives.* As noted by Bradley and Davino (2002) and Henriques and Jones-Brown (2000), incarceration may provide a traumatized woman the time and energy to process life issues, away from parents, partners and the difficult challenges of daily life. Programs were designed/adapted to fit flexibly into a relatively brief time frame.
- *For some women, prison is the safest place in their lives.* It may be the first time in years they are clean of drugs and alcohol in a protected space. That space should remain safe from further trauma, and free of drugs and alcohol. Legislation to make sexual contact with an inmate a felony, video cameras in public areas, and increased contact with community members, actions initiated by the Director, helped to ensure that safety.
- *Programming should be holistic, addressing the range of challenges inmates often face.* Green, Miranda, Daroowalla, and Siddique (2005) identified needs similar to those in our sample: substance abuse, education, job training, parenting skills, domestic violence, sexual assault (psychoeducational), HIV risk, mental health issues. One wing of intensive substance abuse treatment incorporated all these issues in ongoing programming; women living in other wings could elect to attend any of the dozen or so programs offered.
- *It is of utmost importance for everyone working within prison confines to protect inmates' well-being.* Interventions designed to help an individual address difficult past issues may also make them more vulnerable in an environment where ongoing help may not be available. Efforts to increase women's assertiveness may backfire, as COs see her new behavior as defiance and punish her.
- *Inmates are only "in" for a small part of their lives, while they are members of the larger community for most of their lives.* Substance abuse and mental health treatment should be community-based, so that women can continue their services upon release (Vigilante, et al., 1999). Externally based program staff can also avoid role conflicts inherent for some prison personnel (e.g., being required to carry a weapon).
- *Change is not "all or none."* To view a return to prison as "failure" misses small but important incremental changes an individual may have made in their choices and behavior, which over several incarcerations may ultimately add up to the goal of nonrecidivism. The Transtheoretical (Stages of Change) approach (for an overview, see http://www.uri.edu/research/cprc/TTM/detailedoverview.htm), adapted by Jody Brown (1997) for this project, provides a model for evaluating such positive changes.
- *The disconnect between people "inside" and people "outside" needs to be reduced.* Every person who spends time working with inmates is a better-educated person; many gain an understanding they will share with others. Thus the prison should encourage student interns, volunteer programs, and community-based interventions that bring in a wide variety of individuals. A pre-post-discharge mentoring program has helped with the transition back into the community.
- *Prison-based interventions can only go so far in helping women make changes in their lives.* Effective discharge planning needs to address barriers that exist for women on release: homelessness, lack of education and job skills, poverty, ongoing substance abuse treatment, therapeutic interventions for mental illness (Hall, Baldwin, & Prendergast, 2001; Richie, 2001). At the present time, these barriers often prevail over the gains made while in prison.
- *Many offenders now confined in a prison could be better served (and for far less cost) by community based treatment programs.* Residential substance abuse and mental health treatment may be both more effective and cost-efficient (Roskes, Cooksey, Feldman, Lipford, & Tambree, 2005; Tyuse & Linhorst, 2005). RIDOC has initiated a Community Corrections program, but so much more needs to be done here and nationally.

TABLE 1. Contrasting University and Prison Research Settings

University	Prison
Academic freedom	Strict control
Experimental rigor	No control over extraneous environmental factors
Voluntary participation is clear	Inmate is ward of the state, "voluntary" never clear
Subjects typically high functioning	Subjects under stress, vulnerable
Goal is knowledge, publication	Goal is effective management, change
Deliberative publication process, with peer review	Feedback wanted for immediate application to programming
Outcomes help shape future research	Outcomes affect individuals' lives

multiple levels (Stevenson & Ciarlo, 1982). To better inform policy decisions, the evaluation team must try to gain a thorough understanding of the process of service delivery from the outset, and maintain connections throughout the course of the project. Thus, before and throughout the data collection we held extensive meetings with various stakeholders, scrutinized ethical and pragmatic aspects of our goals and procedures, held debriefings with students and amongst ourselves, and discussed our in-depth reviews of and reflections on the research literature. What follows, then, are the issues we confronted, the lessons we learned, and the discoveries we made about ourselves as well as the women we were studying.

TRAUMA IS INHERENT IN CORRECTIONS RESEARCH

We entered this project with trauma in the forefront of our anticipated concerns. First and foremost, we had to be concerned about the welfare of our participants. As other papers in this volume clearly demonstrate, people in the custody of a penal system are multiply traumatized, not only by past experiences, but also potentially within the environment in which they are living and yet again from their partners and others once released. Some may be experiencing continuing traumatic stress because of separation from their children (Enos, 2001), as well as ongoing problems their children or loved ones may be experiencing. Others may be mourning losses of friends and family members who abandoned them because of their problems. A few women first learned they were HIV-infected when they were tested on admission to the prison. Then there are traumas and losses that happen on the outside, such as the death of a loved one. She must watch family and friends going through tough times from afar; rarely would an inmate be allowed to visit a dying friend or family member. We adopted several approaches for this project, starting with educating ourselves and members of our team about trauma and its effects, stressing the need for protection of inmates' well-being above all else, and minimizing the potential for additional trauma created by our own research process.

Our concern about trauma was not limited to the inmates. Anyone who has ever seen a movie set in a prison, watched a news report about prison conditions, or even read the "police beat" in their local newspaper has been exposed to a negative image of criminal offenders and prisons. For those of us who had never been inside a prison, we might as well have been plunging headlong down into the rabbit hole of Alice's Wonderland, and we understood that those we were bringing with us might be frightened as well by this prospect and disturbed by the experiences they were there to learn about. Thus we also discuss here our efforts to prepare for and cope with our own trauma experiences in this project.

Our increased awareness was also motivating, however. We understood that the research we were doing was important. Sadly, without significant levels of intervention, it was unlikely that these high levels of trauma effects would alter upon release back into the community (Bonta, Pang, & Wallace-Capretta, 1995; Weston Henriques & Manatu-Rupert, 2001). If they leave prison with their addictive patterns, abuse vulnerabilities and inadequate job skills intact, at least a quarter of these women can anticipate a quick return to their "ways," with continuing violence from intimate partners and customers alike. While we were not the agents of change, we could provide feedback to help increase program effectiveness, and use our new knowledge to increase public awareness of the need for effective programming for inmates.

PROJECT DESCRIPTION

The project itself focused on structural evaluations of the discharge planning process, as well as quantitative and qualitative data from surveys given at three time points (baseline, shortly prior to release, and 2-3 months post-release) to the incarcerated women. The survey asked about their lives before and since coming to prison, their participation in programs, their perceived readiness to re-enter society and avoid problems upon release, and once released, how they were doing. Over the three years of funding from NIJ, seven faculty members from three academic departments, three members of the prison staff, 13 graduate students, and 30 undergraduate students were active participants in designing and carrying out the project. Several of us spent 1-2 days a week over a period of a year inside the prison interviewing inmates and staff, and collecting survey data on 234 women, 106 of them at two time points and 60 at the third post-release interview.

As stated at the outset, this paper is not the place for reporting statistical results. For our purposes it is sufficient to know that, in line with national statistics (Bureau of Justice Statistics, 2005) many (at least half in most cases) of these women grew up in an abusive, or at best problematic, home; had experienced academic, social, and emotional challenges; did not have sufficient education or job training to obtain regular employment; experienced high levels of adult trauma; and were trying to eke out a life for themselves and their children in spite of habitual problematic substance use, poverty, and a severe lack of resources. The effects of childhood sexual abuse and ongoing trauma overlay these disadvantages in potent and pervasive ways, reducing an inmate's chances of turning her life around as an adult. Most of the women had long ago joined with peers and partners who supported a criminal identity that included sex work and drug abuse (Graham & Wish, 1994). Finally, positive gains made while inside incarcerated could easily be overwhelmed upon release, since many of the women left prison without housing, employment, or effective emotional support.

While we work with group data, we also have tried to see our participants as individual human beings, as members of our community. Establishing rapport with our participants through informal conversations was a transformative experience for each of us, and helped reduce the "us-them" mindset. It also helped us to resist the temptation to classify all of "them" together as one unitary group. Any wing of any prison contains the same rich variety of individuals one finds in any group on the outside. Important differences among subgroups may be found as well; for example, in our sample, Latinas had more educational and health challenges than African-American or European-American women. It is crucial to understand the diverse, and often multiply oppressed, backgrounds of participants and the meanings they have for an individual's situation (Figueira & Sarri, 2002; Primm, Osher, & Gomez, 2005).

CONCERNS, CHALLENGES,
AND CREATIVE (OR SEAT-OF-THE-PANTS) SOLUTIONS

We put on brave faces and adopted an optimistic standpoint that we hoped would (and largely did) come to pass. But in reality, we each brought fears, anticipations of frustration, and many concerns to the project. We were concerned that the confusing, sometimes highly political organizational context would be difficult to work with. As researchers, we bemoaned the limitations on the kinds of questions we could ask (e.g., those which might elicit reports of illegal behaviors while incarcerated or not already part of their criminal record, which might place them in legal jeopardy), the very real possibility that our questions would precipitate painful memories for the women we were wanting to help (see Wincup, 2001), the potential for psychometric inadequacy (few scales have been assessed psychometrically with incarcerated men or women), the need to rely on self-report (no doubt reflecting the larger cultural belief that offenders are unreliable), and the daily "hassles" of doing research in a large institutional setting. As faculty responsible for the well-being of our students, we worried not only about placing young people in situations of potential danger, but also about their emotional well-being after being exposed to lives with such deep trauma. And, frankly, we always worried about one of us doing or saying something that would harm an inmate in some way, even unintentionally.

The students brought their own concerns. Yael Efreom, a senior undergraduate, interviewed some of the students involved in the project for her honors thesis. They shared many of the experiences of the faculty researchers; as one said, "My first day ... I was very scared and nervous but after being thrown into the situation I found the experience greatly boosted my confidence." Interestingly, five of the seven students she interviewed changed their attributions regarding the origins of criminality during the course of the study from dispositional to situational: "My causal explanations did change when I realized the women had experienced so much abuse. Also, the extent of the violence they had experienced and their early exposure to drugs and alcohol definitely made me realize that situational factors were more important" (The other two had begun with situational attributions). All 7 volunteers believed that this experience was highly valuable; five indicated they would like to work with women inmates again.

There were also disparate interests of the staff. Some of the Correctional Officers (COs) were clearly not pleased with potential demands on their time and interruptions of their already-busy schedule. Program staff were concerned that we were there to evaluate them personally, and understandably were worried that a poor evaluation would cost them their contracts with the Department of Corrections Some staff bemoaned having inexperienced and uncommitted (in the sense that we would be leaving within a few months) newcomers interfering with their carefully established relationships with the inmates and potentially "stirring up trouble."

We worked to build a bridge between two systems with widely disparate missions. We chose to acknowledge and address each stakeholder's concerns early and often, and came to realize that our fears, while understandable, could be transformed into understandings that ultimately benefited not only our research process and data quality, but could also potentially clarify and facilitate the way in which business was done at the correctional facility. One example of this occurred in the process of developing a flow chart of the discharge planning process from the time of sentencing to release. Over a pizza lunch (we bought the food), we chatted about their various roles and place within the process. Even as we were constructing the "overflow chart," as we came to describe it, staff began commenting on the disjunctures they were observing through fresh eyes. By the time we had completed our report about a month later, they had recommended–and seen approved–changes that simplified and rationalized the process considerably–a phenomenon known to evaluation researchers as "process utilization." In the same focus groups, some discharge planners noted that they felt that the emphasis on client "success" was unfair. For example, Spanish-speaking inmates participated less often in the English-only programming. As a result, when compared to peers, caseworkers working with these inmates appeared to be less "successful." The other planners agreed to acknowledge this uneven playing field, which they had not previously recognized openly, in future performance evaluations.

Another area where we were able to help them considerably was in database management. When we started, there was no readily accessible database for tracking program participation and other important information. (At that time, data on each new inmate was being kept on index cards in a basement office in another part of the prison.) Our multitalented graduate assistant (KM) stepped forward and volunteered her time to set up a database for program staff (also helpful to our own data collection), which was much appreciated.

Some challenges we had to live with. One particular CO was often rude and caused us delays. We learned to smile and thank her, especially after one of us (KQ), unaware that the room we were waiting in was "bugged," bemoaned the treatment and was made to wait a very long time. Some days a woman we sought for follow-up testing had been released early, moved to another building, or had gone to court. At any time an interview might be interrupted by a "bed check," requiring all inmates to go sit on their cots for counting. One team was caught up in a "lock down" for an hour or so, although their safety was never in question. We came to recognize that what were to us minor inconveniences were, to the inmates, everyday realities that even the kindest staff couldn't always prevent. At any moment they could be demeaned, insulted, relocated to another facility, ordered to move to another cot, strip-searched, or sent into solitary confinement.

ETHICAL ISSUES

We were certainly mindful of the dictum to "first do no harm." We also had a laundry list of ethical codes we needed to follow: the Department of Corrections' (DOC) Code of Ethics and Conduct, the university's Institutional Review Board, NIJ regulations, the American Psychological Association's Ethical Principles of Psychologists, and for the clinicians in our group, the State of Rhode Island Clinical Psychology Licensure codes. We went through several hours of training required by the prison on health and security issues. By law, the prisoner is a ward of the State who forfeits many of her rights while incarcerated. This placed us in a tricky position. While we were presumably more believable because we were from outside the institution, we also wore DOC-issued badges and were obligated to inform officials if we learned or suspected that an inmate might be planning to escape or to harm herself or others. Friendly exchanges with administrators or COs could bring increased credibility or mistrust with inmates, depending on the observer.

We chose to address ethics from the feminist therapy approach elucidated by Laura Brown (1994). We did not stop at the formal requirements, but attempted to proactively identify and address the subtle, implicit issues that might come into play, positively and negatively. Once data collection began, we tried to put safeguards in place to ensure ethical and humane research. By bringing ethical issues into the forefront of training and practice, we felt we could improve not only the experience for our participants, our student assistants, and ourselves, but also for the integrity of our data (see also Fine et al., 2003). Some of the formal and informal issues we identified, and the ways we addressed them, follow.

Educating ourselves and our students. Before we began gathering data, we familiarized ourselves with the situation we were entering; DOC staff (notably RR and JF) were invaluable in helping us prepare for the range of experiences our participants might bring to our interactions. We reviewed the literatures on trauma, substance abuse, and incarceration (e.g., Chesney-Lind, 1997; Harden & Hill, 1998). An expert in corrections Leo Carroll, who had studied this particular prison system (Carroll, 1998) educated us in the political and structural dynamics we might face.

Survey development. Aware that our participants may have difficulties with the typical research format, we wrote our survey and adapted our scales along the lines described by Quina et al. (1999): Consent forms, instructions and items were revised to approximately a 5th grade reading level; response alternatives were clear and easy to mark; and we provided caring, encouraging messages to participants as they moved through more difficult questions. We held focus groups with women in the prison, and revised the survey accordingly.

Informed consent. Each participant needed to feel that her participation was voluntary. This was not always easy. We rewrote the standard informed consent form and trained our assistants to speak in terms the inmate could understand. We explicitly defined our roles, which could easily been confusing to the participants. For example, after our first focus group several women were asking if we were coming back the next week, clearly in anticipation of a therapy group. We had to be very clear about the payment system and to stress that they might not ever be able to earn the payment. Even with these precautions we were always wary of misunderstandings that might arise. Word-of-mouth among inmates can be an ally or deal a devastating blow.

Subtle pressures. At times we noted subtle pressures to participate, or not to participate, from peers, COs, and staff. During the pre-release testing, we would sometimes have to ask the supervising CO to call for a specific woman; the tone of that call ("bark" or "please") could set the tone for the entire interaction and her feelings of safety about it. We could not control backlash from a CO annoyed about having to accommodate space needs, or from fellow inmates who might harass a woman about her participation. On the other hand, a woman who did not respond to a CO's encouragement to participate might experience negative repercussions. We had to rely on the program staff to watch for difficulties when we were not around, and to spot-check with women about their experiences.

Data integrity. No doubt many subtle factors also affected the scope and quality of our data. To a certain extent staff controlled our access to women for interviews; for example, they might discourage us from speaking to those they perceived as emotionally unstable or hostile. We also learned to be patient in soliciting volunteers and ever mindful of the woman's state of mind. Willingness to participate might be dramatically affected by the promise of a new lawyer, a crisis in a family member's life, or a conflict with another inmate; in contrast, long periods of repetitive uneventfulness might translate into disinterest in any activity. "We'll check back" was an oft-used phrase. Several inmates told us that the attitude of caring and respect that we conveyed, even in subtle signals, directly affected their willingness to participate and the integrity of their responses on our survey.

Secondary victimization. We had to be mindful of the effects on ourselves of reviewing traumatic experiences with participants. Secondary victimization effects have recently received some attention (Figley, 1995; Stoler, 2002; Ana Bridges, personal communication, October 6, 2006), and deservedly so. The stories these women told were often wrenching. Nor did the women shy away from their pain, often telling their stories in graphic language and detail. To this day some ring in our ears: the young woman whose first sense of parental approval came at the age of nine when she used drugs with them (and was forced into sex by her father); the street-wise 25-year-old who, reading the item about whether a parent had "threatened you with a weapon" asked us whether a fence post (wielded often by her mother) counted as a weapon. Time spent in the prison was jarringly contrasted with our "free" time; as we exited through electronically locked doors, past razor wire fences, and emerged into bright sunshine. As we drove away, the car became a place where, alone or together, we could allow ourselves to more fully feel the pain we had encountered and to "decompress" before re-entering our more mundane lives. We gave our students and ourselves permission to dissociate from the experience, constructing some psychological walls between our professional time spent within the prison from our personal time outside. We shared strategies with each other, helped considerably by the skilled clinicians (AVG and MG) on our team.

Although we took precautions–undergraduates were paired with graduate students or faculty, and after each session there was an opportunity for debriefing–and although the clinical psychologists on the team provided support for all of us, we found the whole process extremely draining. We were concerned that, following the parallels drawn by Figley (1995), we might ourselves engage in unhealthy cognitive strategies to cope with the experience. We discussed the importance of self-care with our students, and tried to practice it ourselves. We also focused on the positives: we truly felt privileged to be allowed to sit and talk with some very brave women for even this brief time. Ultimately we came to see that our best way of dealing with our sadness was a commitment to making their stories known, transforming them into tools for action.

Respecting boundaries. A related potential for harm was the issue of boundaries. One Sister of Mercy who had worked in the prison for 25 years gave us an extraordinary gift of her insight about how women in prison have had to learn how to please others in order to survive. This was not a warning to mistrust them, but rather a "heads-up" regarding the potential for harmful dynamics, either by reinforcing their willingness to help us in ways that crossed boundaries, or by tapping into their attempts to please by pushing for participation when they would rather not do so. We had to learn to monitor our reactions and our behaviors: to step back from our egos when we were feeling charmed, to make explicit our boundaries and observe them, and to be mindful about our motives in every interaction.

Staying within our role. We also were often tempted to provide comfort beyond the normal expressions of concern or support, to give advice, or even suggest alternative ways of living their lives (so easy for us to see, it seemed!). We stressed to participants that we were not there as therapists or to offer programs, and worked to avoid even the slightest hint of judgmentalism in our conversations. Recognizing that our survey might leave some respondents uncomfortable or sad, at the end of each interview we offered the participant a chance to talk about it, expressed our own caring concern, and then reminded them of resources within the prison system (social workers, and program staff who other inmates had indicated were trustworthy and helpful) to whom they could talk. If we were concerned about a participant's distress or safety, or felt we had not handled a situation as well as we might have liked, we discussed it with the appropriate staff person (usually the social worker). At the same time, acutely aware of the limited access to individual therapy,[2] we tried to avoid actions that might distress the inmate.

Compensation. It bothered us that we were asking so much of these women for so little in return. For a variety of reasons, the only offer we could make was $25 in cash if they took the two-month post-release survey, and then only if they were out of the prison at that time. (Fewer than a third of the 106 women who qualified at pre-release could be found on the outside to take us up on that offer.) We knew that it was difficult for them to work through a tedious survey, twice, being asked very personal questions, and were already sensitive to the pressures they might be under to participate. However, that fear was unfounded. Indeed, the women thanked us for our time, for caring enough about them to come and do the study. They appreciated our efforts to evaluate the programs so that they might continue to be offered. At a more personal level, they appreciated that we cared enough about them to let them tell us their story. We came to realize how rarely those of us on the outside even think about those on the inside, and how seldom they experienced someone from outside sitting down and making them feel they have something to offer. From this grew an increasing sense of responsibility to personally honor their trust in us, as well.

Security. We had to develop a complex strategy for handling data. We obtained appropriate federal and state assurances regarding protection of individual responses from external review. All team members were instructed in issues of confidentiality. We developed complex double-coding systems, kept surveys with us when we left the prison, and acquired a locked file cabinet onsite for follow-up survey information. We kept a notepad (also locked up) which allowed us to track what had been done, who had asked us to come back the next day, and so on, but made sure no personal information (other than the name and a brief message) was written down.

Privacy. Privacy can be tricky to achieve in a prison setting. Imagine a large central "recreation room" with a dozen or so women milling about playing cards, watching television, or chatting. Interruptions were common, as friends might stop by and even ask, "what did you say on that question about ..." At times we were seated uncomfortably close to a CO or one might walk by regularly. Even low-tone discussions could potentially be overheard. Decisions about whether to continue an interview had to be left to the discretion of the participant and the researcher in the moment. To their credit, team members managed to obtain a substantial number of fully completed surveys; once word got around that we were "ok people" our participation rates were boosted by encouragement from other inmates.

Fatigue. We had planned to conduct qualitative interviews at the end of each survey. These tended to be brief and unproductive, turning instead into more general chatting about the participant's life, or her view of the study. The women seemed tired of answering formal questions, and obviously enjoyed an opportunity to interact with someone "from outside." Since this was the part of the experience that participants and researchers enjoyed the most, we quickly gave up the idea of qualitative data collection and encouraged the conversations, as long as they did not cross boundaries. Ultimately, the impressions the participants made on our team members during these conversations were among the most lasting benefits of the entire experience.

CONCLUSIONS

We had set out on a journey to learn about the impact of discharge planning programs on women being released from prison. But those of us usually working within the framework of academia or clinical practice learned so much more. We developed a respect and admiration for the women we interviewed, often an awe for the survival skills they had developed. We learned to let go of the "tyranny of empiricism," and listen to what they were teaching us. Our collaborators, the prison administrators and staff, also learned that observant outsiders could help them streamline and enhance their own procedures.

Research with an incarcerated population requires constant care and attention to everyone's best interests, an ethics that goes beyond the formal rules and permeates the attitudes and behaviors of the research team. There are no simple answers to the issues we have raised here, nor were our solutions the only or necessarily best ones. When being ethical conflicts with being efficient, or getting "good" data, ethics must win.

Such research also requires that we learn about a large institutional system and adapt to it. It requires that we be sensitive to the "inmate" and "researcher" roles we bring to the situation, as well as the immediate and personal experiences of the participant. We demonstrated this could be done, in spite of the controlled and starkly "enclosed" nature of this environment. And we learned that while an invasion of researchers can be informative for the "insiders," it is even more transformative for the "outsiders."

The expectations we entered with were not the understandings we left with. We did not anticipate how impressed we would be by these women, and how much we would admire their skills as competent survivors of an unforgiving world; yet that was the most salient thing our experiences left us with. We have tried to maintain that awareness as we discuss our work with others, acknowledging at all times the humanity of the women we came to admire and respect.

If asked "would you do it again?" the answer would be a resounding "yes!" We would encourage others to do more research or to provide interventions with incarcerated populations. Beyond that, we would encourage readers to not forget the people who spend part of their lives beyond the bulletproof glass.

AUTHORS NOTE

The authors were a collaborative; as such, the author order is for convenience and does not differentiate among contributions, which were numerous from each member. The authors thank Leo Carroll, Jennifer Morrow, Cheryl Hevey, and Yael Efreom for their work on this project. The authors would also like to thank the women who participated in this study, anonymously, but each leaving a special impact on our lives.

This research was supported by National Institute of Justice grant #96-CE-VX-0012: "Collaborative Development of Individual Discharge Planning for Incarcerated Women" (1/1/97-12/31/98, extended to 12/31/99).

NOTES

1. Since the project ended, Warden Richman has become Assistant Director of Rehabilitative Services, responsible for many departments of RIDOC including Community Corrections. Some of these programs have not been continued.

2. Mental health counseling was not regularly available, and as in many systems, *pro bono* work was not allowed because of union restrictions. AVG was able to set up a student training practicum, and anger management programs are still in place at a men's federal detention center in Rhode Island.

REFERENCES

Bonta, J., Pang, B., & Wallace-Capretta, S. (1995). Predictors of recidivism among incarcerated female offenders. *Prison Journal, 75*, 277-294.

Bradley, R., & Davino, K. M. (2002). Women's perceptions of the prison environment: When prison is "the safest place I've ever been." *Psychology of Women Quarterly, 26*(4), 351-359.

Brown, J. (1997). Working toward freedom from violence. *Violence Against Women, 3*(1), 5-26.

Brown, L. S. (1994). *Subversive dialogues: Theory in feminist therapy.* New York: Basic Books.

Bureau of Justice Statistics (2005). *Prison statistics.* Retrieved 10/1/06 from http://www.ojp.usdoj.gov/bjs/prisons.htm.

Carroll, L. (1998). *Lawful order: A case study of correctional crisis and reform.* New York: Garland.

Chesney-Lind, M. (1997). *The female offender: Girls, women, and crime.* Thousand Oaks, CA: Sage Publications.

Enos, S. (2001). *Mothering from the inside: Parenting in a women's prison.* Albany, NY: State University of New York Press.

Figley, C. R. (Ed.). (1995). *Compassion fatigue: Coping with secondary traumatic stress disorder in those who treat the traumatized.* NY: Brunner/Mazel.

Figueira-McDonough, J., & Sarri, R. C. (Eds.). (2002). *Women at the margins: Neglect, punishment, and resistance.* Binghamton, NY: The Haworth Press.

Graham, N., & Wish, E. D. (1994). Drug use among female arrestees: Onset, patterns, and relationships to prostitution. *Journal of Drug Issues, 24,* 315-329.

Green, B. L., Miranda, J., Daroowalla, A., & Siddique, J. (2005). Trauma exposure, mental health functioning, and program needs of women in jail. *Crime & Delinquency, 51*(1), 133-151.

Hall, E. A., Baldwin, D. M., & Prendergast, M. L. (2001). Women on parole: Barriers to success after substance abuse treatment. *Human Organization, 60*(3), 225-233.

Harden, J., & Hill, M. (Eds.). (1998). *Breaking the rules: Women in prison and feminist therapy.* New York: The Haworth Press.

Henriques, Z. W., & Jones-Brown, D. D. (2000). Prisons as "safe havens" for African American women. In M. W. Markowitz & D. D. Jones-Brown, (Eds.), *The system in Black and White: Exploring the connections between race, crime, and justice* (pp. 256-273). Westport, CT: Praeger.

Primm, A. B., Osher, F. C., & Gomez, M. B. (2005). Race and ethnicity, mental health services and cultural competence in the criminal justice system: Are we ready to change? *Community Mental Health Journal, 41*(5), 557-569.

Quina, K., Morokoff, P. J., Harlow, L. L., Deiter, P. J., Lang, M. A., Rose, J. S., Johnsen, L. W., & Schnoll, R. (1999). Focusing on participants: Feminist process model for survey modification. *Psychology of Women Quarterly, 23*(3), 459-483.

Richie, B. E. (2001). Challenges incarcerated women face as they return to their communities: Findings from life history interviews. *Crime & Delinquency, 47*(3), 368-389.

Roskes, E., Cooksey, C., Feldman, R., Lipford, S., & Tambree, J. (2005). Management of offenders with mental illnesses in outpatient settings. In C. L. Scott & J. B. Gerbasi (Eds.), *Handbook of correctional mental health* (pp. 229-257). Washington, DC: American Psychiatric Publishing.

Stevenson, J., & Ciarlo, J. (1982). Enhancing the utilization of mental health evaluation at the state and local levels. In J. Stahler & W. Tash (Eds.), *Innovative approaches to mental health evaluation* (pp. 367-386). New York: Academic Press.

Stoler, L. (2002). Researching childhood sexual abuse: Anticipating effects on the researcher. *Feminism & Psychology, 12*(2), 269-274.

Tyuse, S., W., & Linhorst, D. M. (2005). Drug courts and mental health courts: Implications for social work. *Health & Social Work, 30*(3), 233-240.

Vigilante, K., C., Flynn, M. M., Affleck, P. C., Stunkle, J. C., Merriman, N. A., Flanigan, T. P., et al. (1999). Reduction in recidivism of incarcerated women through primary care, peer counseling, and discharge planning. *Journal of Women's Health, 8,* 409-415.

Weston Henriques, Z., & Manatu-Rupert, N. (2001). Living on the outside: African American women before, during, and after imprisonment. *Prison Journal, 81*(1), 6-19.

Wincup, E. (2001). Feminist research with women awaiting trial: The effects on participants in the qualitative research process. In K. R. Gilbert (Ed.), *The emotional nature of qualitative research* (pp. 17-35). Boca Raton, FL: CRC Press.

doi:10.1300/J229v08n02_08

Index

Note: Page numbers followed by the letter "t" designate tables; and numbers followed by the letter "b" designate boxes.